Advance Praise for
The Yamas & Niyamas...

"Beyond moral precepts, the yamas and niyamas are guidelines for living a healthy life. With the voice of a storyteller, Deborah Adele brings this ancient wisdom to light with modern tales common to us all. This is the behavior we need for a sustainable world."

> ~ Anodea Judith, Ph.D., www.SacredCenters.com
> Author of *Eastern Body-Western Mind* and
> *Waking the Global Heart*

"The Yamas & Niyamas is a great book. It is one that I have been looking for, for a long time. Deborah's style is fresh and truthful, her writing inviting and inspiring, and her suggestions for integrating the concepts into life - downright simple. You'll learn a lot from this book and along the way you'll have fun exploring yourself."

> ~Susi Hately Aldous, BSc., yoga teacher, founder
> of Functional Synergy Yoga Therapy and author of
> *Anatomy and Asana* and *The Art of Slowing Down,*
> www.anatomyandasana.com

"After reading *The Yamas & Niyamas: Exploring Yoga's Ethical Practice*, I wanted to return all my other books to the shelf and just practice these teachings. The insights that Deborah Adele draws from yoga's ethical guidelines have helped me to better understand my Christian faith. I am buying a copy of this book for each and every member of my prayer groups."

> ~ Rev. Douglas Dirks, Abilene, Texas

"Compassionate, lively, and wise, *The Yamas & Niyamas* provides a portal into a recognition beyond tradition; a living way to relate from our highest vibratory level into our present world, regardless of cultural or religious background. Like the Tao expresses itself as yin and yang, these restraints and observances are presented as the swinging doors into the unconditional, liberating us from the bonds of our day to day stressors and uniting us with the One truth for which we all hunger. It fed me."

~ Randine Lewis, MSOM, L.Ac., Ph.D.
Founder of The Fertile Soul, www.thefertilesoul.com
Author of *The Infertility Cure* and *The Way of The Fertile Soul.*

"Deborah's book, *The Yamas & Niyamas: Exploring Yoga's Ethical Practice*, really brings these jewels to the light and to the world. As a yoga teacher I have been looking for something for my students that can lead them to join me in a life-long love affair with the yamas and niyamas – and this is it!"

~ Dharmi Cunningham, owner Turning Light Studio,
N. Yarmouth, Maine, www.turninglight.org

"Deborah Adele has written a jewel of a book. In this volume, we find not only the practical insights of classical yoga, but simultaneously the deep wisdom, subtlety, and joyfulness that these practices produce. *The Yamas & Niyamas: Exploring Yoga's Ethical Practice* is a must read for anyone interested in spiritual wisdom."

~ Phil Nuernberger, Ph.D., www.mindmaster.com
Author of *The Warrior Sage* and *Strong and Fearless:
The Quest for Personal Power*

THE YAMAS
&
NIYAMAS

THE YAMAS

&

NIYAMAS:

Exploring Yoga's Ethical Practice

by Deborah Adele

On-Word Bound Books, LLC
publishing & media ~ Duluth, Minnesota

THE YAMAS & NIYAMAS: Exploring Yoga's Ethical Practice
Copyright © 2009 by Deborah Adele

Published by:
On-Word Bound Books LLC / 26 East Superior Street #402
Duluth, Minnesota 55802 / www.onwordboundbooks.com

Fonts: Main text: Adobe Garamond Pro. Titles and quotes: Shangri La and Rowen Oak by Nick's Fonts http://www.nicksfonts.com/

Haiku's written by Catharine Larsen

Sanskrit resources were found on-line at the following websites:
http://learn-sanskrit.com:80/8limbs.htm
http://www.avashy.com/hindiscripttutor.htm
http://www.americansanskrit.com
Sanskrit was illustrated by Sara Duke and approved by Vyaas Houston of the American Sanskrit Institute.

Library of Congress Cataloging-in-Publication Data

Adele, Deborah, 1949-
  The yamas & niyamas : exploring yoga's ethical practice / by Deborah Adele.
     p. cm.
  ISBN-13: 978-0-9744706-4-1 (pbk.)
  ISBN-10: 0-9744706-4-3 (pbk.)
  1. Yoga. 2. Ethics. 3. Conduct of life. I. Title. II. Title: The yamas and niyamas.
  BJ123.Y64A34 2009
  181'.45--dc22

                              2008032793

Printed in the United States of America
10 9

Dedicated to:

Yogiraj Achala
who made these ten guidelines come alive in my life,
and to all sentient beings
whom I hope will benefit from this exploration.

Acknowledgments

A book is never written in a vacuum; I have been humbled by this truth. To all of those whose participation made this book a reality, my deepest love and gratitude; your voices are contained within these pages as well as in my heart.

Deepest gratitude to the sages and teachers who sit within the yogic tradition, whose selfless sharing of the richness of the yogic tradition with the West has brought a new sense of awareness, balance, and opportunity to Western consciousness. My prayer is that we in the West are worthy of the gift and can use this wisdom for the broader scope of humanity and the earth.

Deepest gratitude to Yogiraj Achala whose love and teaching have given me pieces of myself.

Deepest gratitude to Vyaas Houston of the American Sanskrit Institute for his generous guidance crafting Sanskrit characters. His character is impeccable and his love for Sanskrit is both moving and inspiring. Please check out the opportunities available to you at www.americansanskrit.com.

Gratitude to Catharine Larsen for sharing her insights and creativity in the beautiful Haikus which begin each chapter. The book is richer for them.

Deepest gratitude to my friend and business partner Ann Maxwell, who embodies these guidelines. Although the words of this book are mostly mine, they come from our work together over our years as business partners and represent the thoughts and experience of both of us. Throughout the book you will hear the purity of her voice and the boldness with which she lives her life. We have a partnership that we have consciously chosen to base on practicing these guidelines with one another; this choice has kept us fresh and pertinent.

Gratitude to Jill Pospisil whose support, editorial comments and tireless research gave clarity and integrity to this book. Gratitude to Phil Nuernberger, Ph.D., whose constant support and encouragement kept me on task; Phil has been a significant teacher in my life. Gratitude to the Rev. Douglas Dirks, Dharmi Cunningham, and Ron Johnson who were kind enough to read, encourage, and give direction to the pages of this book; their willingness and love was a strong foundation and impetus for writing.

Thank you to Brooks and Coral Anderson who generously provided rustic cabin space on Lake Superior where the silence could render the writing of this book. Thanks also to Nancy Hanson-Bergstrom and John Bergstrom, Catharine and Lauren Larsen and to Ron Johnson who shared their homes as writing space for me.

Thank you to the publishers, Sara Duke and David Devere, whose clarity, ideas, and love of books kept me encouraged and inspired. They have made this process a fun and creative adventure; I am grateful that they took the risk.

Thank you to Michelle Skally Doilney and Debbie Nuernberger, who gave me permission to shut my door and write.

Gratitude to the amazing community of people who practice and learn at Yoga North Studio in Duluth, Minnesota; their strong dedication and commitment has deeply touched my heart.

Gratitude and love to my family and friends who provide the venue for living the practice of these guidelines and love me anyway.

And finally, deepest love and gratitude to my husband, the Rev. Doug Paulson, whose tireless nourishment, love, and support is beyond words. Doug continues to stimulate my thinking, model a selfless life, encourage my explorations, provide humor to the monotonous, and make every day a grand adventure. ࿊

Table of Contents

Preface

I have a favorite mug that sits on my office desk filled with pens and pencils. This mug was given to me by one of my brothers many years ago, and I still look at it daily and chuckle. The mug says:

Things to do today:
1. Stop the Arms Race
2. Floss

I mention the mug because not only does it keep me tuned to both the lofty ideals of my life as well as the practical components, but it also speaks to the essence of the *Yamas & Niyamas*. These ten guidelines sit as both a vision of the possibilities of human existence, as well as providing the practical guidance to make skillful moment to moment choices in our daily lives.

We all want to live well. Let's face it, at the end of the day, it's not how much you have or how much you have accomplished that counts. What matters is how well you have participated in your own life, both the ordinary routines and the extraordinary surprises. It's how you feel inside when you lay your head on the pillow. Does a feeling of joy and well-being accompany you to bed? Or does your head touch the pillow with thoughts of anger, bitterness, helplessness, frustration, self-disappointment, or whiny complaints?

Being human is a complicated thing. We live within myriad confusing choices and contradictions. As human beings living among other life forms, we need to navigate our own personal needs within those of the community. As

Spirit hanging out in a human body, we need to live within the potential of our limitless dreams and our limited physical reality. In the midst of our indecision and confusion, these guidelines are like helping hands moving us deeper into our own authenticity and into a life that is richer and fuller than we could ever imagine, simply because we are living with more skill and awareness.

This may sound easy, but it is not. How do we gain mastery over our choices when life seems to toss us around with its ups and downs, many demands, and many voices telling us what we need and what is wrong with us? How do we gain skill when we find ourselves continuing to do what we promised ourselves we would never do again? How do we gain skill when we just screamed at our child or our partner and now we feel lousy? How do we gain skill when we feel stuck in a dead end job that is sucking us dry? How do we gain skill when we just dug into the chocolate and now we are beating ourselves up with messages of self-loathing?

Gaining the skill to choose our attitude, to choose what we think, and to choose what we do, may be the grandest adventure we can take as a human being. In the film *Last Holiday* Georgia Byrd, shocked by discovering she has only three weeks to live, decides to make her dream life of possibilities into reality. In an amazing shift of character from a timid woman stuck in her perceived realities of life, she suddenly bursts forth boldly and claims the life she has always wanted for herself.

It doesn't need to take a death sentence for us to change. We have the choice to burst forth boldly and claim our lives in this very moment, and yoga's ten guidelines, the *Yamas*

& *Niyamas*, can support that very leap into the life that we seek. Under their guidance, the turbulence and drama that are often a familiar part of our life begin to disappear.

The result of a skillfully lived life is nothing less than joy. Not the kind that comes when things are going our way and disappears just as quickly, but the kind that bubbles up from within. The kind of joy that comes from our own sense of mastery in life that no matter what life brings, we are ready. Maybe there is nothing to figure out ahead of time, there is only a life to live well...or not. Which are you choosing for yourself? ❧

What are the Yamas & Niyamas?

The *Yamas & Niyamas* are foundational to all yogic thought. Yoga is a sophisticated system that extends far beyond doing yoga postures; it is literally a way of living. Yoga is designed to bring you more and more awareness of not only your body but also your thoughts. The teachings are a practical, step-by-step methodology that bring understanding to your experiences, while at the same time pointing the way to the next experience. They are like a detailed map, telling you where you are and how to look for the next landmark. They facilitate taking ownership of your life and directing it towards the fulfillment that you seek.

The *Yamas & Niyamas* may be thought of as guidelines, tenets, ethical disciplines, precepts, or restraints and observances. I often think of them as jewels, because they are the rare gems of wisdom that give direction to a well-lived and joyful life. In yogic philosophy, these jewels sit as the first two limbs of the 8-fold path.*

The first five jewels are referred to as *Yamas*, a Sanskrit word which translates literally into the word "restraints" and includes nonviolence, truthfulness, nonstealing, nonexcess,

---

*The 8-fold path, or Astanga Yoga, comes from the Yoga Sutras of Pantanjali. Pantanjali, curious about what held true for all the different kinds of yoga, codified these basic tenets of all yoga in writings called the Yoga Sutras. Our word suture comes from the same word; think of these truths as weaving your life together in much the same way a medical suture would thread your torn body together. The writings of the Yoga Sutras form a basic text for classical yoga. The other six limbs of the 8-fold path are *Asana*, or postures; *Pranayama*, or breath control, *Pratyahara*, or sense withdrawal; *Dharana*, or concentration; *Dhyana* or meditation; and *Samadhi*, a state of unity.

and nonpossessiveness. The last five jewels are referred to as the *Niyamas*, or "observances," and include purity, contentment, self-discipline, self-study, and surrender. Many guides to ethical conduct may leave us feeling overwhelmed with concepts, or boxed in by rule sets. Yoga's guidelines do not limit us from living life, but rather they begin to open life up to us more and more fully, and they flow easily into one another in ways that are practical and easy to grasp.

Nonviolence, the first jewel, sits as the foundation to the other guidelines, which in turn enhance the meaning and flesh out the richness of nonviolence. Nonviolence is a stance of right relationship with others and with self that is neither self-sacrifice nor self-aggrandizement. This tenet guides us to live together, share the goods and do what we want – without causing harm to others or ourselves.

Truthfulness, the second jewel, is partnered with nonviolence. The marriage of these two guidelines creates a powerful dance between two seeming opposites. We can appreciate this statement when we begin to practice speaking our truth without causing harm to others. As partners, truthfulness keeps nonviolence from being a wimpy cop-out, while nonviolence keeps truthfulness from being a brutal weapon. When they are dancing perfectly together, they create a spectacular sight. Their union is nothing short of profound love in its fullest expression. And when there is cause for disharmony or confusion between the two, truthfulness bows to nonviolence. First and foremost, do no harm.

Nonstealing, the third jewel, guides our attempts and tendencies to look outward for satisfaction. Often, our dissatisfaction with ourselves and our lives leads us to this outward gaze, with a tendency to steal what is not rightfully ours. We steal from the earth, we steal from others, and we steal from ourselves. We steal from our own opportunity to grow ourselves into the person who has the right to have the life they want.

Nonexcess, the fourth jewel, has been interpreted by many to mean celibacy or abstinence. Although this could certainly be one interpretation of nonexcess, its literal meaning is "walking with God." Whatever your beliefs about the Divine, this tenet implies an awareness of sacredness in all our actions and an attentiveness to each moment that moves us into a stance of holiness. From this place of sacredness, the boundary is set to leave excess behind and live within the limits of enough. If we have been practicing nonstealing, we will automatically find ourselves primed to practice this guideline.

Nonpossessiveness, the fifth jewel and last of the guidelines known as the *Yamas,* liberates us from greed. It reminds us that clinging to people and material objects only weighs us down and makes life a heavy and disappointing experience. When we practice letting go, we move ourselves towards freedom and an enjoyment of life that is expansive and fresh.

If we have begun to live the first five jewels well, we may notice that our time is freeing up and there is more breathing space in our lives. The days begin to feel a little lighter and easier. Work is more enjoyable and our relationships with others are a little smoother. We like ourselves a little more; there is a lighter gait to our step; we realize that we need less than we previously thought; we are having more fun. As we begin our study of the final five jewels or *Niyamas,* we move into a more subtle realm and into an interior resting place, a place that becomes like Sabbath for us.

Purity, the sixth jewel, is an invitation to cleanse our bodies, our attitudes, and our actions. It asks us to clean up our act so we can be more available to the qualities in life that we are seeking. This precept also invites us to purify how we relate to what is uppermost in the moment. It is the quality of being aligned in our relationship with others, with the task at hand, and with ourselves.

Contentment, the seventh jewel, cannot be sought. All the things we do to bring fulfillment to ourselves actually interfere with our own satisfaction and well-being. Contentment can only be found in acceptance and appreciation of what is in the moment. The more we learn to leave "what is" alone, the more contentment will quietly and steadily find us.

Self-discipline, the eighth jewel, literally means "heat" and can also be translated as catharsis or austerities. It is anything which impacts us to change. Change makes us spiritual heavyweights in the game of life; it is preparation for our own greatness. We all know how easy it is to be a person of high character when things are going our way, but what about those times life deals us a dark card? Who are you in those moments? This guideline is an invitation to purposefully seek out refining your own strength of character and it asks, "Can you trust the heat? Can you trust the path of change itself?"

Self-study, the ninth jewel, is a pursuit of knowing ourselves, studying what drives us and what shapes us because these things literally are the cause of the lives we are living. Self-study asks us to look at the stories we tell ourselves about ourselves and realize that these stories create the reality of our lives. Ultimately, this tenet invites us to release the false and limiting self-perception our ego has imposed on us and know the truth of our Divine Self.

Surrender, the tenth jewel, reminds us that life knows what to do better than we do. Through devotion, trust, and active engagement, we can receive each moment with an open heart. Rather than paddling upstream, surrender is an invitation to go with the underlying current, enjoy the ride, and take in the view.

In this book, each *Yama & Niyama* has been given its own chapter in which the philosophy of the guideline is woven with practical examples and stories. At the end of the chapter, I've included a list of questions as a guide for reflection. I encourage you to journal and/or form a study group to help deepen your commitment to your learning and to yourself. ෨

AHIMSA

Storms rage about me.
I calm my heart and send out
ribbons of peace ~ peace.
~ C.L.

अहिंसा

Ahimsa: Nonviolence

In the *Karate Kid* movies, Mr. Miyagi at first appears to be a silly, rather harmless little old man to seventeen year old Daniel. Mr. Miyagi is humble and unpretentious; he sits around for hours trying to catch flies with chopsticks, tends his bonsai trees, and doesn't even seem to bat an eye when provoked. But as the movie progresses and bullies threaten both Daniel and Mr. Miyagi, Mr. Miyagi springs into defensive action. Daniel's eyes are opened to the incredible ability of this old man who skillfully takes on a team of karate opponents larger and younger than he is. From that point on, Mr. Miyagi becomes Daniel's mentor in the art of skillful defense, true friendship, and the art of living.

Nonviolence may appear to us like Mr. Miyagi first appeared to Daniel. It can look so passive and unimportant that we can easily ignore its presence and the subtleties of its power, wondering what the fuss is all about. And yet, in Eastern thought, nonviolence is so valued that it stands as the very core and foundation of all yoga philosophy and practice. It is as if the yogis are saying that if we don't ground our lives and actions in nonviolence, everything else we attempt will be precarious. All of our achievements and successes, hopes and joys stand on faulty ground if they do not stand on the foundation built by nonviolence.

> In Eastern thought, nonviolence is so valued that it stands as the very core and foundation of all yoga philosophy and practice.

Killing and doing physical harm are grosser forms of violence that are easily seen and understood. However, nonviolence has many subtle implications as well. When we feel hurried, afraid, powerless, out of balance, and harsh with ourselves, we may find ourselves speaking words of unkindness or even exploding with a violent outburst. As our awareness of these nuances grows, we learn that our ability to be nonviolent to others is directly related to our ability to be nonviolent within ourselves. Our inner strength and character determine our ability to be a person of peace at home and in the world.

In the *Karate Kid* movies, Daniel did not go to karate school to study. Instead, he became skilled at karate by learning how to move through the daily chores of waxing cars, sanding wood, and painting fences. In much the same way, we grow our capacity to be nonviolent by learning how to move through the everyday challenges of life and by addressing the things that precipitate our tendencies toward violence. *Ahimsa*, or nonviolence, literally to do "no harm," calls forth from us our most brilliant and best self. Our capacity to be nonviolent depends on our proactive practice of courage, balance, love of self, and compassion for others.

Finding our Courage

We only have to look around us to see that fear abounds. It abounds in cowardly faces that turn away, in violent attacks, in walls of protection, in bins of possessions, in numerous unkind words and gestures. In an abundant world, hoarders take more than their share leaving others lacking. Wars are started and fought to seize the goods and keep the power. All around the world, children's innocence is destroyed by abuse and horror. If we look closely, we can trace all of these acts of greed, control, and insecurity back to their root: fear. Fear creates violence.

If we are to begin to address these fears, we need to know the difference between the fears that keep us alive and the fears that keep us from living. The first kind of fear is instinctual and built in us for survival. The second kind of fear is fear of the unfamiliar. The unfamiliar can become an abundant place for our exploration once we realize this fear lives only in our imagination. It is only our minds that have created the turmoil in our gut and kept us hostage to the possibility of our own lives.

An example of fear that lives only in the imagination, might be sky diving. For me, the thought of jumping out of a plane at a high altitude and remembering to open my parachute somewhere along the way, sends cold shivers down my spine and giant rumblings of fear in my gut. All of this is happening in my body in this very moment, and yet I have never experienced this activity. For me to walk into this fear, I would first imagine a different scenario for myself, something that looks like adventure and fun; something where I am competent

> To create a life and a world free of violence is first and foremost to find our own courage.

and collected as I jump from heaven to earth. And then, were I really to step into my courage, I would call a pilot.

Seeking out people and experiences we would normally avoid provides a fertile place to learn new things about ourselves and about life. Even those we might call enemies have much to teach us. People we have previously avoided will open up new ways of thinking and will give us pieces of ourselves. As we walk into our fears with both people and experiences, we will find that our sense of self has grown. Our view has expanded; the world suddenly looks like a bigger place, and we are more competent to navigate in it. As we expand ourselves into these new places, our minds and hearts grow more open and we have less need to be violent. Thus, to create a life and a world free of violence is first and foremost to find our own courage.

Courage is not the absence of fear, but the ability to be afraid without being paralyzed. Courage is found by facing our fears – the small ones, the fat ones, the embarrassing ones, and the really big, scary ones. To live the fullness that our own life is inviting us into, we often have to let ourselves be afraid and do it anyway. If we keep ourselves safe, how will our courage grow? One of the reasons for Gandhi's unmatched power was that he continued to stay with life; he didn't run when life got too confusing or difficult. He stayed and learned from the moment, and in the process he became a skillful leader no one could match and a force that no one could stop. For Gandhi, fear became a stimulus to develop his courage.

Creating Balance

Courage demands our best self and that is a self in balance. Think about the times you were "short" with others because of too much work to do, or too much caffeine and sugar, or a restless night of sleep. Imbalance in our systems is almost a certainty for violence, as the "dis-ease" we feel within finds its way to expression outwards. Balance creates harmony within

अहिंसा

us, and harmony within naturally expresses itself in external actions that are harmonious. Dr. Phil Nuernberger emphasizes the importance of balance when he says, "The deep harmony of balance is my most precious commodity and I guard it fiercely."

Creating balance in our lives is not an easy thing. We are a hungry, noisy people, bombarded with stimulation and advertisements that promise to grant us our deepest desires. If we are not on purpose with creating balance for ourselves, we can easily fall victim to false promises and fill every breathable space with appointments and activities and all the responsibilities that go with a full agenda. It is anti-cultural to claim any space that is simply space, or to move with any kind of lingering, or to take time for closure. We are bombarded and we bombard ourselves. And if we have any doubts, our calendars will reveal the truth of our craziness. The repercussions are inescapable, immeasurable violence to ourselves and those around us.

> Balance comes from listening to the guidance and wisdom of the inner voice.

Like the body, the mind and soul need time to digest and assimilate. Like the body, the mind and soul need time to rest. We create this rest by allowing space that we can breathe in. Not more clutter, but more space, space to reflect, space to journal, space for closure, space for imagination, and space to feel the calling of the life force within us.

Balance does not look a certain way because it isn't a set standard to impose upon ourselves; it's not something we can plan or schedule. Balance instead comes from listening to the guidance and wisdom of the inner voice. Balance will look different in each of us and even different in each of us at different times. To be in tune with ourselves, we must get quiet and listen and then heed this inner voice. This voice does not push or bombard or make promises. This inner wisdom simply knows what we need to be vital, healthy, and in deep harmony.

My sons and their children love the board game Risk. It is a game where all the players begin with armies, which they strategically place on various countries around the world, and then try to conquer the world with their armies. It is a game of strategy and skill and can be played into the wee hours of the night. What is interesting to me is that my grandchildren, in playing this game, have learned something important about balance. One of my grandchildren put it this way, "When you see someone's army spread all over the world, it looks so impressive. Dad always starts by putting all his armies on four countries in a corner. It looks like no one will ever have to worry about him. But as the game gets played, the person who has spread their armies too thin is always the first to lose, and Dad always wins."

> When we are in balance, we automatically live in nonviolence.

Balance is like this. Spreading ourselves thin looks impressive, but in the end, we are the first to lose. The health and well-being of our body, mind, and spirit is a powerful resource and by keeping ourselves in balance, we can stride through life with greater competence and ease. We are primed to "win" as we meet life from an inner place of harmony. When we are in balance, we automatically live in nonviolence.

Powerlessness
Dealing with Powerlessness

One of the biggest challenges to maintaining balance is feeling powerless. Feeling powerless leads to outward aggression in the form of frustration and anger, or withdrawal inward into depression and victimization. We fear our own power and we often feel trapped at our sense of powerlessness. By powerless, I mean those times we feel like we've run out of choices. We've run out of options and we are feeling totally incompetent to deal with the challenge at hand. At these times, we may feel like a caged animal, trapped and ready to spring. Whether we respond with anger, withdrawal, frustration, or resignation, there is a way in which our mind shuts down, as if we are riding a train through a dark tunnel and we can't see anything but darkness and anxiety.

Ahimsa, or nonviolence, invites us to question the feeling of powerlessness rather than accept it. When we feel powerless, we have forgotten how much choice we really have. We have a choice to take action and we have a choice to change the story we are telling ourselves about our powerlessness. Instead of sulking in the feeling of powerlessness, we can ask, "What do I need to do right now to feel competent to handle this situation?" During these times, we can also jumpstart ourselves by remembering past times when we successfully handled a challenging situation while remaining loving and whole and then trying to find that feeling again.

I have found three ways of thinking that shift me out of a feeling of powerlessness: practicing gratitude, trust in the moment, and thinking about others. When I change my approach, I am out of the dark tunnel of powerlessness. Suddenly, in the light, I see many options. For instance, if my car breaks down at an inconvenient time, I can choose to be grateful that I am safe and have my cell phone; I can choose one of many options for support for towing and fixing my car; I can turn the whole situation into an adventure by perhaps riding the bus for the first time in years or calling an old friend for a lift, and trusting that somehow, all is well.

Often we carry a sense of powerlessness from a childhood story. Perhaps at one time in our lives, the story was true, but it probably isn't true anymore. I do many private consultations with people who are feeling powerlessness from believing an old story that they have continued to accept as true. I have come to believe that any sense of powerlessness we are feeling can be traced back to the story we are telling ourselves in the moment about the situation. We all have the choice to tell a different story and grow ourselves up to take responsibility for our lives in a new and fresh way.

> One of the biggest challenges to maintaining balance is feeling powerless. Nonviolence invites us to question the feeling of powerlessness rather than accept it.

Situations where we feel powerless can also be opportunities to grow our skill level with life. I find my powerless issues arise with technology and mechanics. When things break down, my feelings of powerlessness can become a violent outburst or an opportunity to learn something new.

I often ponder the words of Yogiraj Achala, "I excite myself with my incompetencies." With this attitude, feelings of powerlessness become opportunities to become competent rather than violent.

Self-Love

Our ability to stay balanced and courageous has much to do with how we feel about ourselves. The following two stories illustrate this point. Pandit Rajmani Tigunait, spiritual head of the Himalayan Institute, tells of an incident with his young son. The family had just returned from India and the child began behaving strangely. He was biting and pinching his parents and playmates. Rajmani was beside himself with this strange behavior from his sweet son, until he realized that in India his son had gotten worms and the worms were pinching and biting his little insides. The son was only displaying outwardly the experience of his insides.

Yoga instructor and mentor Ann Maxwell tells of the abrupt turbulence in her home when her three year old son, Brooks, suddenly began holding his stools. Holding his stools caused him great discomfort and in turn the whole household was affected to the extent that the day was shaped for the whole family by whether Brooks was releasing or holding his stools. The days he held it in were the days that the whole family suffered from the oppressive misery of a little three year old boy. Brooks was displaying outwardly the experience of his insides.

These stories show that how we treat ourselves is in truth how we treat those around us. If you are a taskmaster with yourself, others will feel your whip. If you are critical of yourself, others will feel your high expectations of themselves as well. If you are light hearted and forgiving with yourself, others will feel the ease and joy of being with you. If you find laughter and delight in yourself, others will be healed in your presence.

We would never purchase a can of red paint and expect it to be the color blue when we apply it to our walls. And yet we can be so harsh and demanding with ourselves and then expect to be loving with others. It just doesn't work that way. The color of the paint inside the can is the color that whatever we paint becomes. The "color" of how we treat ourselves is the "color" of how we treat others. If we can't be safe with ourselves, others can never be safe with us, and the world can never be a safe place to be.

> How we treat ourselves is in truth how we treat those around us.

I spent three years consulting with a firm out of Boulder, Colorado. The work itself was stimulating and rewarding, but I was on such a fast-paced track that one day I realized I had not even taken time in those three years for one of my most delicious pleasures, a long, hot bubble bath. When I finally took a pause to look at the whirlwind life I had created, I also realized I had not played with my grandchildren or checked in with my friends, and I was becoming quite demanding of those around me. Others were feeling my bite. I had created a violent inner world of pushing, overdoing, and under-sleeping that had seeped into all my relationships. When I quit the work and began to bring some ease and pleasure back into my life, all my relationships became more enjoyable and ease filled.

One experiment I did as I began to make this huge change was to practice falling in love with myself. I say experiment because I was curious what affect this would have on others as well as on me. Falling in love is such a delightful place. The other can do no wrong. The loved one is always beautiful and delightful to be with, and you want to be with them all the time. Falling in love leaves no room for the violence of expectations and judgments; it is free for delight and joy and spontaneity. Everyone around the lover also feels the love. Love creates a spontaneous combustion that includes all in its path. Have I succeeded in my experiment? Not entirely, but those who know me report that I am easy and delightful to be with.

We can have hearts that are full of love for others, and intentions to love that are pure. But the truth is, we will express that love for others by treating them the same way we treat ourselves. Love lies at the core of nonviolence and begins with our love of self. Not a love that is ego-centric but a love that is forgiving and lenient; a love that sees the humor in the imperfections and accepts the fullness of the human expression. Only when we find this love for all the parts of ourselves, can we begin to express fully the love that wells up inside of us for others. Finding this love for all the parts of ourselves means we have to forgive ourselves. Without forgiveness, we carry guilt like a heavy burden around our hearts. Guilt holds our love for self and others hostage and keeps us bound to a one-sided expectation of the human experience.

I cannot say this enough times. Our inability to love and accept all the pieces of ourselves creates ripples—tiny acts of violence—that have huge and lasting impacts on others. I have, in my life, the privilege to hear many people speak their personal feelings, and I am constantly surprised by how much of their speech is a reporting of failings and self-loathing, and attempts to "fix" themselves. These attempts to change self, rather than love self, keep us trapped in vicious cycles that we can't crawl out of. There is such a big disconnect for me as I hear others share their personal confessions of failure. Even as I hear the words, I am seeing before me a beautiful, unique expression of the human being and my heart is overwhelmed. And I find myself once again uttering my secret prayer that this person could someday see how magnificent they really are.

Courage and love are deeply connected. "When love became the Lord of my life, I became fearless." These words were expressed by Swami Rama in his journey on this earth and are echoed by Jesus' statement, "Perfect love casts out fear." Where fear creates harm and violence, love creates expansion and nonviolence and the true safety that we seek. Nonviolence is woven with love, and love of other is woven with love of self; these cannot be separated.

Violence to Others

If we cannot find love for our self, it becomes easy to look outward and begin to focus on others, hiding our own sense of failure and fear under our blazing concern for others. It's almost as if we are secretly saying, "My life is a mess; I'll feel better if I fix yours." If we are not honest with ourselves, we can even go to bed with a sense of pride in the amazing things we have done for others that day. We may even feel holy about our arduous feats of self-sacrifice. In reality we are hiding our own sense of self-failure by telling others how to live their lives.

When we are unwilling to look deeply and courageously into our own lives, we can easily violate others in many subtle ways that we may not even be aware of, thinking that we are actually helping them.

Thinking we know what is better for others becomes a subtle way we do violence. When we take it upon ourselves to "help" the other we whittle away at their sense of autonomy. Nonviolence asks us to trust the other's ability to find the answer they are seeking. It asks us to have faith in the other, not feel sorry for them. Nonviolence asks us to trust the other's journey and love and support others to their highest image of themselves, not our highest image of them. It asks that we stop managing ourselves, our experience, others, and others' experiences of us. Leave the other person free of our needs, free to be themselves, and free to see us as they choose.

> When we are unwilling to look deeply and courageously into our own lives, we can easily violate others in many subtle ways that we may not even be aware of, thinking that we are actually helping them.

The violence we do to others by thinking we know what is best for them is dramatically illustrated in a story from India. It seems a passerby witnessed a monkey in a tree with a fish. The monkey was saying to the fish, "But I saved you from drowning!" The monkey, thinking it had saved the fish, had taken the fish to a place that couldn't meet any of the fish's needs for survival or growth. We can't save people, or fix them.

All we can do is model, and that points the finger back at us.

I experienced this well-intentioned "help" from my husband who, out of love for me, began to take anything heavy out of my arms and carry it himself. At first I thought this was sweet of him and appreciated the gesture, but over a period of time I began to notice that some of the strength was leaving my arms. By not occasionally carrying heavy things, I was getting weaker!

Handling challenges gives each of us a sense of skill, self-esteem, and accomplishment. When we try to fix or save someone else, we are keeping them from getting the learning the situation has for them. Like the monkey in the story above, when we try to take someone out of their challenge or suffering, we take them out of the environment that offers them a rich learning experience. We are in a sense, cutting them off from the power of growing stronger, more competent, and more compassionate.

It can often feel like torture to let a person we care about sit in the suffering and challenges of their life. We almost can't help ourselves; if they are hurting we want to make them feel better. If they have a decision to make, we want to tell them how to make it. And yet, the only thing we have to offer that is truly of value is to sit with them, where they are, as they are. We need to trust suffering and trust challenge and trust mistakes; they are what refine us when we don't run from them.

Nelle Morton, a feminist writer of the '70s spoke eloquently about the power we have to "hear each other into being." Rachel Naomi Remen echoes, "Our listening creates a sanctuary for the homeless parts within another person."

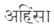

There is nothing to fix or save in another; there is only the gift of listening. People need a safe place to "hear themselves." To return to the monkey and the fish story, all we have to offer in the end is to get into the water with those in need, not to bring them into the tree with us.

Worry is another way violence gets masked as caring. Worry is a lack of faith in the other and cannot exist simultaneously with love. Either we have faith in the other person to do their best, or we don't. Worry says I don't trust you to do your life right. Worry comes from a place of arrogance that I know better what should be happening in your life. Worry says I don't trust your journey, or your answers, or your timing. Worry is fear that hasn't grown up yet; it is a misuse of our imagination. We both devalue and insult others when we worry about them.

I'd like to discern the difference between *help* and *support*. For me, *help* carries the connotation that I am more skilled at life's decisions and challenges than the other person is. *Help* is a "one up" on the other person. Whereas *support* meets the other person on equal playing ground with equal ability and is able to sit with more awe and respect than answers. The Chrysalis Center for Battered Women in Minneapolis, Minnesota has a beautiful motto that embodies the concept of trusting over worry and support over help. The motto states, "Every woman has her own answer. Every woman has her own timing. Every woman has her own path."

It comes down to this: Do I go to my child, my friend, my partner, myself, with love or with worry? Which has more breath, more space, more efficient use of energy, more building power? What would happen in the lives of others if we could choose love over worry and carry this kind of trust and belief in our loved ones. When we can truly love and accept all of our self, compassion begins to blossom in our hearts, and we begin to see others with different eyes.

Developing Compassion

We learn compassion as we dissolve our personal version of the world, and grow gentle eyes that are not afraid to see reality as it is. We learn compassion as we stop living in our heads, where we can neatly arrange things, and ground ourselves in our bodies, where things might not be so neat. We learn compassion as we stop trying to change ourselves and others and choose instead to soften the boundaries that keep us separated from what we don't understand. We learn compassion as we do simple acts of kindness and allow others' lives to be as important as our own.

When we begin to expand the boundaries of our heart, we can see clearly to act in ways that truly make a difference. Compassion is a clear response to the needs of the moment. We see this truth lived out in the lives of the great ones. They act with a compassion and skill that truly changes things.

In the New Testament, the Greek word that gets translated into compassion is *splagchnizomai*. This word literally means to have feelings in the bowels or other inward parts. We tend to think of the heart as the place of compassion, but in Jesus' day, emotions were understood to be centered in one's bowels. Because compassion was understood to carry a very visceral, gut wrenching, inner reaction, it was used sparingly by the New Testament Gospel writers. When the Gospel writers did use this word, it was to portray a person that was touched so deeply and profoundly by the situation of another, that they were moved to take immediate action on behalf of the one who was suffering. These Gospel writers understood compassion to be more than a sorrowful feeling; it was a powerful inner response leading to an immediate outward action that took a risk on behalf of the other.

> We learn compassion
> as we dissolve our
> personal version
> of the world,
> and grow gentle eyes
> that are not afraid
> to see reality
> as it is.

A friend tells of an incident that happened to her many years ago. A woman with a new baby from the apartment next door began frantically screaming that her husband had locked himself in the bathroom and was killing himself. My friend, after dialing 911, broke all the rules of keeping herself from danger by somehow getting into the bathroom and beginning to hold this man who was by now lying on the floor bleeding profusely. My friend risked all precautions to soothe and comfort this man as they both waited for help to come.

Compassion is like this. It moves us across the boundaries of established norms and often past the boundaries of safety, rushing headlong to do what it can to ease another's suffering. Compassion forgets itself and the standards of protocol to answer the cries of another. We may not yet have the kind of courage and depth of compassion that my friend displayed, but we can, in all of our encounters, begin to practice acts of kindness.

When my husband was eleven, his dad was killed in a car accident, leaving seven small children and a stunned wife behind. My husband continues to tenderly tell and retell how one of his uncles began to periodically stop by the house, coaxing himself and his siblings into the backyard for a game of softball, taking them to their very first Viking football game, and on the best of snow days, driving them to a secluded road with a fabulous hill. From there the uncle would haul them in his station wagon up the hill so that they could ride their sleds down that hill, only to repeat the action again and again. Seeing seven bewildered nieces and nephews, whose father had been suddenly killed, this uncle had compassion. No one had asked him for anything. This uncle, moved by a visceral gut feeling, took unsolicited action on behalf of the whole family. It made all the difference for my husband.

Lucille Clifton once said, "Every pair of eyes facing you has probably experienced something you could not endure." Every human being walking this earth has painful stories tucked in the corners of their hearts. If we could remember this truth, perhaps we could see with the eyes of compassion rather than the eyes of our own judgments and preferences.

While attending a workshop at Esalen, I met a man from Tokyo who epitomized the compassion and gentleness of nonviolence. He had a certain light about him, and I observed that others were as attracted to him as I was. I was delighted one afternoon to find myself in his company during lunch and being privileged to hear his story. He had been on the fast track in Japan, an entrepreneur of great talent and dedication, moving up the success ladder at a rapid pace. In one swift moment his life changed when his best friend, who had been paralleling this life of high success, suddenly dropped dead of a heart attack.

I sat mesmerized as this man across from me at the table, spoke in low and certain tones that at that moment he saw his life unfold before him and instantly retired from business to begin running marathons. More incredibly, he had never trained. He just began to run for the love of running and for the love of life. Now in his late 40's, he has been running a marathon a week for the past five years. To look at him, I had to marvel because he had a stocky body with bowed legs. And yet, he had never suffered even the slightest injury. He flew all over the world to run a marathon a weekend and that was his training. When asked how he accomplished this kind of stamina with no injury and no training, he reverently replied, "With each step I touch the earth lightly to do her no harm, and she in turn does me no harm."

Whatever we find ourselves engaged in, this jewel of *Ahimsa,* or nonviolence, asks us to step lightly, do no harm, and to honor the relationship we have with the earth, with each other, and with ourselves. ☙

Questions for Exploration

Living with these questions, taking time for reflection, and journaling will give you new insights into your life and the practice of nonviolence. For this month, frame your exploration in the following statement by Etty Hillesum, a young holocaust victim:

Ultimately we have just one moral duty:
to reclaim large areas of peace in ourselves,
more and more peace,
and to reflect it towards others.
And the more peace there is in us,
the more peace there will also be in our troubled world.

Week One: This week practice courage by doing one thing daily that you wouldn't normally do. If you're feeling brave, make that one thing something that scares you. If you're feeling really courageous, get excited about the fact that you're scared and you're doing it anyway. See if you can discern between fear and the unfamiliar. Watch what happens to your sense of self and how your relationships with others might be different because you are courageously stepping into unknown territory.

Week Two: This week guard your balance as you would your most precious resource. Don't find your balance from a place in your head of what it should look like. Instead, find guidance from the messages of your body. In this moment do you need more sleep? More exercise? Do you need to eat differently? Do

you need to pray? Do you need some variety in your life? Act on the messages of your body and explore what balance looks like for you this week. Notice the effects on your life and on others.

Week Three: This week, watch where you are running interference on others' lives. Are you a worrier? A fixer? Discern the difference between "help" and "support." Notice what you might be avoiding in your own life because you are so interested in others' lives.

Week Four: For this whole week, pretend you are complete. There is no need to expect anything from yourself or to criticize or judge or change anything about you. No need to compete with anyone, no need to be more than you are (or less than you are). Note your experience. Notice how much pleasure, kindness, and patience you can allow yourself to have with yourself.

For this month, ponder the words of Etty Hillesum and bring more and more peace inside you. ೞ

SATYA

*Is my "yes" coming
from a dark corner or from
the light in my heart?
~ C.L.*

सत्य

Satya: Truthfulness

Perhaps you have read *The Chronicles of Narnia* by C.S. Lewis. This delightful series has certainly been a favorite in my family over the years. In a passage from the first book of the series, *The Lion, the Witch and the Wardrobe*, four children are about to be introduced to the mighty King Aslan by Mr. and Mrs. Beaver. Mr. Beaver lets them know that Aslan can right wrongs, banish sorrow, drive out winter and bring spring to the land. When asked if Aslan is a man, Mr. Beaver sternly declares to the children that Aslan is definitely not a man – he is the King of Beasts and anyone who approaches him should go with their knees knocking. The children are afraid that Aslan isn't safe and their fears are confirmed by Mr. Beaver. But he also assures them that, although the King of Beasts isn't safe, he is good.

Like Aslan the lion king, the jewel of *Satya*, or truthfulness, isn't safe, but it is good. Truth has the power to right wrongs and end sorrows. It is fierce in its demands and magnanimous in its offerings. It invites us to places we rarely frequent and where we seldom know what the outcome will be. If we don't approach truth "with our knees knocking," we haven't really understood

> The jewel of *Satya*, or truthfulness, isn't safe, but it is good.

the profoundness of this guideline. We may think that truth means simply not fibbing to our mom when she asks if we ate the forbidden cookie. But truth demands integrity to life and to our own self that is more than not telling a simple lie.

When we are real rather than nice, when we choose self-expression over self-indulgence, when we choose growth over the need to belong, and when we choose fluidity over rigidity, we begin to understand the deeper dynamics of truthfulness, and we begin to taste the freedom and goodness of this jewel.

Be Real Rather than Nice

Carl Jung writes, "A lie would make no sense unless the truth was felt to be dangerous." Why do we lie? Are we afraid to hurt someone's feelings or afraid if we told the truth we would not be liked or admired anymore? I have a friend who says, "I pick the right-sized box, put myself in it, wrap it with pretty paper and a bow, and then 'present' myself to the other person." I have another friend who states, "I always show up differently with different people. My biggest fear is that everyone I know will be in the same room at the same time and I won't know who to be."

> My biggest fear is that everyone I know will be in the same room at the same time and I won't know who to be.

And then there is the whole topic of "nice." I once heard Yogiraj Achala say that you have to watch out for nice people. Being a nice person myself, I was at first offended and then confused, so I took this statement to heart and began pondering its truth. I began to see the distortion that sits between nice and real.

Nice is an illusion, a cloak hiding lies. It is an imposed image of what one thinks they should be. It is a packaging of self in a presentable box, imposed by an outer authority. People who are "nice" hold truth inside until they reach a breaking point and then they become dangerously inappropriate; I know because I used to be such a person.

Real comes from the center of our unique essence and speaks to the moment from that center. Real has a boldness to it, an essence, a spontaneity. Real asks us to live from a place where there is nothing to defend and nothing to manage. It is a contact with the moment that is not superimposed or prepackaged. Real is something we might not always like in another, but we come to know there will be no surprises. Real, though not always pleasant, is trustworthy. When I met my husband, I mistook him for a gay man. As a result I didn't display myself as I normally would have if I had thought there might be a chance for romance. I know now that the deepness we have in our relationship has been built from the foundation of that first experience of showing him the real, authentic me. And he in turn, has given me the same gift of realness.

What is driving you to distort yourself or silence yourself or say yes when you mean no? Or as Carl Jung would ask us, what is so dangerous in the moment about the truth that you are choosing to lie? These are questions that merit our pondering.

Self-Expression vs. Self-Indulgence

When we habitually silence and distort ourselves, we begin to lose our lust for life and look towards other things to fulfill us. We forget that we are here on this earth to self-express in a way no one else ever has or ever could. We can feel this urge within us wanting to bubble up and say to the world: I'm here! Our self-expression can find its way into the world in many forms, but when the process of our self-expression is imposed on for whatever reason, we can easily turn towards self-indulgence. Most often this imposition comes in the form of *should's* or *should not's*, either from our own self messages or from others' messages to us. The result is always a misdirection of energy. There is a settling for less than we had hoped for, a kind of resolution to things as they are. Often we find ourselves hiding by overeating or overworking, rather than doing what we really want to do.

> Living the life that cries to be lived from the depth of our being frees up our energy and vitality. We benefit and everyone around us benefits.

Living the life that cries to be lived from the depth of our being frees up a lot of energy and vitality. The juices flow. Everyone around us benefits from the aliveness that we feel. On the other hand, suppressing that life, for whatever reason, takes a lot of our life energy just in the managing of the pretending.

Arthur Samuel Joseph, nationally known voice teacher and author of the book *Vocal Power: Harnessing the Power Within,* gives his first time students an interesting assignment. He tells them to go home and record themselves reciting a poem and then singing a song. Then he tells them to take off all their clothes and repeat the exercise. Joseph says that when the student returns for their next lesson and presents their homework, Joseph can always tell which recording was done naked because the "naked" version is much more vibrant.

In all the ways we package ourselves and protect ourselves, or when we choose the safety of belonging over the inner need to grow we also dull ourselves.

The Need to Belong vs. the Need to Grow

In the Family Constellation work of Bert Hellinger (therapeutic work dealing with family systems), a unique slant on guilt and innocence is expressed. Hellinger says that as human beings we have both a need to belong to groups and a need to expand and grow. Hellinger says that as long as we stay within the approval of the group, we experience the innocence of belonging. However, when we begin to grow in directions beyond the group, we experience guilt in regards to the group. The truth of our freedom carries the price of guilt.

I experienced this in my own life when I embraced feminism. At that time, feminism was a refuge for me that gave voice to many of the experiences of my life. It just made sense to me that women were as important as men and that there should be equality between the sexes. My mother was mortified because feminism went against everything she believed in; I couldn't have done anything more evil in her sight. I found myself feeling guilty in relationship to her

> Human beings have both a need to belong to groups and a need to expand and grow.

and the love I felt for her, and yet I knew that for that time in my life I was following a deep longing in my soul. Although our love for each other remained strong and intact, my choice around feminism remained a painful topic for both my mother and me.

The groups we belong to are many: our country, our culture, our gender, our class, our age group, our race, our religion, our family of origin, our community, our workplace, and the various organizations that we are members of. All these groups have rules and belief systems, some written, some silently understood, that must be followed for us to be part of the group. These rules and belief systems are necessary, they are what shape the group and give the group its identity. As long as these rules don't conflict with our inner longing to grow more and more into our full self, there is no problem. However, when a conflict arises between the need to belong and the need to grow, we have to make a choice. We must either sacrifice a part of ourselves to maintain our belonging, or we must risk the approval and support of the group by growing.

> Truth rarely seems to ask the easier choice of us.

Think of the protestor whose conscience opposes a war her country is engaged in. Following her realness, will she take a stance, even if it means going to jail? Or think of the man who finds himself in a dead-end job that holds no interest or life for him, and yet he has a family to support with kids ready for college. Will he make the switch to a job that excites him but pays a significantly lower salary? Or the young mother who is longing to go back to school but is deeply entrenched in a family and community that demands that mothers stay home and care for their small children. Will she choose the realness of her longing, trusting she can care for her children even more deeply from a place of satisfaction and the excitement of her own life?

In all of these situations, there is no wrong or right choice. Rather, these situations point out why listening to and acting on our inner voice to change and grow, to move on, to speak truth to ourselves and then act on it, can be so difficult at times. If we pursued any of these stories in more depth, we would see that other factors can easily be pulled in as additional reasons to remain in the status quo, stacking the deck even more in favor of staying the same. I often hear people say, "I just don't know what to do." I think more often than not, we do know what to do; the cost of our realness just seems too high at the time.

Truth rarely seems to ask the easier choice of us. In the moment to moment details of our daily living truth asks us to pay attention and to act correctly the first time.

Do It Right the First Time

Yogiraj Achala makes the statement that it is worth the effort to do the task right the first time, because cleanup takes so much time. Think about this for a moment. How much time do you spend having to find someone you were a little harsh with and apologize? Or go back and tell someone you can't really do what you said you would do? Or maybe you spend your time and energy trying to avoid that person because of your own embarrassment. Can you imagine speaking and acting so correctly that you never have to go back and apologize or make a new agreement? Or how much time do you spend avoiding things you dislike, like writing your will or facing your finances? These are all acts of cheating truth that result in messes we eventually have to clean up.

And what about those lies you tell yourself? I continuously find myself in trouble because I lie to myself about time. I make promises to myself and others that don't allow for the reality of interruptions, rest, or play. Then I either have to backtrack on my promises or find myself out of balance keeping up with the too many commitments I have made because of my dishonesty with myself. I also lie to myself when I set

> Can you imagine speaking and acting so correctly that you never have to go back and apologize or make a new agreement?

lofty goals that are more wishful thinking than anything the reality of my days can incorporate. And then I have to clean up the mess I have made with myself. Not only that, but I have become, once again, a person who cannot trust herself.

Can you trust yourself? Can you risk telling yourself the truth? Can you keep the promises you make to yourself and to others? We must be willing to take the risk to tell ourselves the truth and grow ourselves into someone who can trust themselves. We will then be able to easily bear others' trust in us. Being truthful with ourselves makes us trustworthy and frees up all the time we normally spend in guilt and regret from our dishonesty. Truth saves us from having to clean up, and as a bonus, we get to learn something in the process.

"Doing it right the first time" does not always look the same way. Truth is a dance where the rules and certainties change with the circumstances. This fluidity is what makes truth so interesting.

Truth is Fluid

Because of its marriage to nonviolence, truth has a fluidity about it. In one situation truth shows up boldly and courageously, as when we do a tough intervention on a loved one who is faltering under alcoholism. In another situation, truth shows up in a most gentle way, as when we heap praise upon a young child's diligent artwork. Both of these examples show the different flavor that the practice of truth takes when it is partnered with the love of nonviolence. The compassion of nonviolence keeps truthfulness from being a personal weapon. It asks us to think twice before we walk around mowing people down with our truth, and then wonder where everyone went.

The fluidity of truth also requires that we clean our lens, and periodically get new glasses with which to observe the world. Our seeing is limited by all the groups that shape us, as well as by our experience. What we believe, whether we are aware of that belief or not, informs everything we do

> The compassion of nonviolence keeps truthfulness from being a personal weapon.

and every choice we make. To be a bold person of truth is to constantly look for what we are not seeing and to expose ourselves to different views than the ones we hold sacred. As Yogiraj Achala reminds us, "What are you not seeing because you are seeing what you are seeing?"

Carl Jung understood the fluidity of truth when he made the statement that what is true at one time for us, at some point no longer serves us, and eventually becomes a lie. He understood that truth changes over time; what was true when we were two years old is no longer true or even relevant when we are seventeen. In *Modern Man in Search of a Soul*, Jung writes, "Thoroughly unprepared, we take the step into the afternoon of life; worse still, we take this step with the false presupposition that our truths and ideals will serve us as hitherto. But we cannot live the afternoon of life according to the programme of life's morning – for what was great in the morning will be little at evening, and what in the morning was true will at evening have become a lie." The guideline of truthfulness asks us to update our beliefs and values and views in order to stay current with ourselves and our surroundings.

In India, the fluidity of truth was understood in the practice of what was called the *Ashramic Stages*. Life was divided into four equal parts, or times in life, in which a certain aspect of living was honored and pursued. In the first period of life, it was time to grow up and, with the support of your parents, learn a skill in which you showed interest and ability. In the second period of life, it was time to use this skill for the good of the community and to receive money in return so you could live and raise a family. In the third period of life, it was time to leave worldly possessions and tasks in pursuit of inner wisdom. And in the last phase of life, it was time to return to the community, guiding and supporting the community with the inner wisdom that had been attained.

Today's times may feel more complicated to us, but there is something to learn from these *Ashramic Stages*. We can use these stages to ask ourselves if we are engaged in the truthful pursuit that is right for this time of our lives and to assess if we have done something significant to mark these rites of passage. Ritual helps us to end and begin again, without carrying the dead weight of what we have left behind. My oldest granddaughter just marked a turning point when she, along with her whole senior class, met the evening before the beginning of their senior year to write their names in chalk on the high school parking lot. It was a significant event that marked the beginning and ending of a phase of life.

Truth has Weight

Although truth prefers fluidity to rigidity, it also has real substance to it. There is a thickness or a weight to a person who practices truthfulness. I remember hugging my business partner Ann one day and telling her that she was thick. She looked a little taken aback until I explained that I could feel the depth of her integrity and her boldness to make contact with life however it comes to her. I remember literally being able to feel this thickness to her. I could feel her realness. Like Ann, a person of substance is willing to stay present in life no matter what its initial unpleasantness. They know that staying present with the truth of the moment will add more depth to their lives and grow them up to be creative and responsible versus becoming a person who walks around with a subtle "rescue me" sign.

When we run from life, try to manage life, or leave our energy scattered here and there, we feel differently than when our whole self shows up with our thoughts, words, and actions congruent and unified. When we are centered in the moment, we can fully meet the ordinariness of life as well as the challenges of life. Dishes are met with the same contact as are arguments as are hugs. There is no need to tame ourselves or hide ourselves. "All of us" shows up to the moment, ready to meet it in truth and integrity, ready to make full contact. Meeting the moment "full on" is like playing a contact sport. We aren't afraid to play the game with everything we have or to get knocked around a little in the process; it's all part of the fun.

There is a profound courage to this kind of willingness to be raw with reality as it is, rather than to run from it or construct a barrier to soften it. When I traveled to Central America in 1988 with the Augsburg College Center for Global Education, I saw first hand this kind of willingness to be raw with reality, no matter how horrible. At that time, El Salvador was a dangerous place to travel as untold thousands were being picked up, tortured, and disposed of in a state park by the El Salvadoran militia. I sat with mothers of the disappeared whose photo albums showed pictures of their dead loved ones displaying myriad signs of torture. And yet I witnessed courage, love, joy, and community like I have never come close to experiencing since. There was something in the fierceness of the way the people met the truth of their lives and risked for the sake of

> There was something in the fierceness of the way the people met the truth of their lives. They were able to contact life in its fullness.

justice. In a place and time of the greatest of personal horrors, they were able to contact life in its fullness. It was a profound time for me.

I was shocked when I returned to the states from my time in Central America. Everything felt protected and stale to me. It was as if we as a culture have constructed barriers to tame reality. It was as if we as a culture aren't able to risk telling ourselves the truth. Not long ago, I witnessed the pathos of a situation in which a Pit Bull killed a small dog. A few days later my son was in a pet store and overheard the manager tell one of the new clerks that in order to sell the Pit Bull puppy they had in the store the clerk was to tell customers that the puppy was an American Terrier. This effort to construct barriers to hide truth seems to me like a contagious disease in our country. What are we so afraid of?

> What are we so afraid of? What might my life look like if I were willing to contact truthfulness in every moment?

The Power of Truth

One of the things that amazed me when I first read Gandhi's autobiography was his statement about his life being an experiment with truth. I would have expected him to say an experiment in nonviolence, but he didn't – he said truth. To me, this statement captures the power that living with truth has. A poor, colonized country united in nonviolence gaining its freedom; a dominant country brought to its knees. This was arguably the greatest nonviolent revolution in history, and all because of one man's experiment with truth.

It makes me wonder what my life might look like if I were willing to contact truthfulness in every moment. ⟡

सत्य

Questions for Exploration

Living with these questions, taking time for reflection, and journaling will give you new insights into your life and the practice of truthfulness. For this month, frame your exploration in the following statement by Mahatma Gandhi:

> *I know that in embarking on nonviolence*
> *I shall be running*
> *what might be termed*
> *a mad risk.*
> *But the victories of truth*
> *have never been won without risks.*

Week One: This week observe the difference between "nice" and "real." Notice situations where you were nice. What did this experience invoke in you? What were the results? Notice situations where you were real. What did this experience invoke in you? What were the results? From whom or what do you seek approval? Does this affect whether you act from your "niceness" or your "realness"?

Week Two: Spend this entire week in self-expression. Make movement towards the external world with your internal hopes and dreams. Act on life-giving opportunities, despite the consequences. Observe what happens in you. Observe how others react. If you find yourself in self-indulgence, ask yourself, "What am I not expressing?"

Week Three: This week pay attention and go slow enough that you "do it right the first time." Make this a week where you don't have to backtrack to apologize or correct mistakes and where you don't run from any hard tasks that present themselves. Face each moment head on with clarity and courage.

Week Four: This week, look at ideas and beliefs that once served you and now have become archaic. You may unknowingly be holding on to things that you no longer need. Honor these beliefs because, like a vehicle, they brought you to your current place on your journey. As you let go of what no longer serves you, pay attention to where denial shows up and celebrate your movement toward a clearer, more authentic you! Watch how this exercise frees up your energy for the further emergence of your authentic realness.

For this month ponder the words of Mahatma Gandhi and the risks he was willing to take in his experiments with truth. How much are you willing to risk for the victories of truth? ✍

ASTEYA

Why steal from your life
by steeling your will? Instead,
be still and love God.
~ C.L.

अस्तेय

Asteya: Nonstealing

I was recently at a wedding where I had the opportunity to speak with the priest who was officiating at the service. Trying to make conversation, I asked him if, in all his many years of several hundreds of weddings, he had ever had the experience of a wedding being halted at the last moment. He relayed the following story.

It seems that the day of the wedding, the bride-to-be discovered that her almost husband had slept with the maid of honor the night before. She didn't tell anyone about this discovery, but proceeded to prepare for the wedding as normal, walk down the isle, and stand at the altar. The service proceeded up to the point in the ceremony where the Priest asked if there was anyone who objected to the marriage. At this point, the bride spoke, saying, "Yes, I have an objection. I can't in good faith marry a man who would steal from our future together with his actions of last night." She then proceeded to walk down the aisle and out of the church, leaving a stunned groom at the altar and a silent crowd in the church pews.

> *Asteya,* or non-stealing, calls us to live with integrity and reciprocity.

Like the bride in the story above, the third jewel, *Asteya,* or nonstealing, calls us to live with integrity and reciprocity. If we are living in fears and lies, our dissatisfaction with ourselves and our lives leads us to look outward, with a tendency to steal what is not rightfully ours. We steal from others, we steal from the earth, we steal from the future, and we steal from ourselves. We steal from our own opportunity to grow ourselves into the person who has a right to have the life they want.

Stealing from Others

An outward focus leads us to compare ourselves to others and to send our energy into their lives in unhealthy ways. When we compare ourselves to others, we either find ourselves lacking, which makes us feel somehow cheated, or we find ourselves superior, which leaves us feeling somewhat arrogant. Our attention on others from a place of discontent within ourselves can lead us to live vicariously through others or to try to control, manipulate, or manage them in order to boost our own sagging ego. We may find ourselves trying to "trump" or "one-up" their stories and successes and experiences by coming behind them with our own more fabulous tale. It is all an attempt to make ourselves feel better about ourselves.

> When we compare ourselves to others, we either find ourselves lacking, which makes us feel cheated, or we find ourselves superior, which leaves us feeling arrogant.

Perhaps someone is sharing their excitement about an upcoming trip. To which we immediately pipe in with a much more exotic trip that we have planned, or maybe we say that we have already been where they are going. Either way the conversation becomes about us and our trip and we have stolen their excitement about their own trip. We do the same with others' successes. We can even do it with death. For example, if someone's mother has passed, and we shift the conversation to our story of losing our own mother we are making the situation about us, instead of being present for the other person.

Or perhaps we steal from others by not paying attention to them or discounting them. In all the instances where we steal, we have made the situation about us, not about the other. Whatever words have or haven't come out of our mouth, the intent has been to serve ourselves, not the other. When we feel unhappy with ourselves or our lives, we have a tendency to drag people down with us or make snide comments that come from jealousy. When we are genuinely caring of the other, that caring finds expression in ways that feel supportive and tender to the other.

When I was training with Yogi Bhajan, he used to say, "Be a forklift; you should always be lifting people up." The question we can ask ourselves in our encounters with others is, does the other person feel uplifted and lighter because they have been with us, or do they feel like something precious was taken from them? Have we brightened their day by taking a moment to listen, to sincerely compliment them, or simply to smile?

Stealing from the Earth

Not only do we steal from others, but we steal from the earth. We forget that we are spirits having a human experience. We are visitors to the human experience; we are visitors in the fullest sense of the word. You wouldn't go to a friend's house for dinner, complain about the food, leave your trash lying around, and walk off with the candlesticks because you wanted them. And yet, this is so often how we treat our world.

We are visitors to this land, to our bodies, to our minds. To fully appreciate this reality is to accept that nothing on this physical plane does or can belong to us. To "own" something then, becomes a form of stealing. We use the term "I," "mine," and "my" with almost everything… my house, my car, my clothes, my kids…we even say, "I had a flat tire." The ownership of things is steeped deep in our language and culture and makes it hard for us to appreciate the extent to which nothing really is ours. This guideline asks us to view everything in our possession as something precious that is on loan to us. And for the time that it is on loan to us, we are asked to care for it.

> Imagine what would happen if each time we took something, we gave something back.

On this globe there is an increasing gap between those who have and those who do not have. It would be ludicrous for us to think that things could be or even should be evenly divided on this earth, but there is something wrong when children starve and elders wander homeless. Theologian Walter Brueggemann writes that the bounty of the earth is for the community, not the individual. I often wonder what the world would be like if we understood this profound statement and lived as if everything we now think of as "mine" could be used for the good of the community.

Nonstealing implies more than not taking what isn't ours. It is an inherent understanding that from the moment we are born, we are in debt to this gift called life. The ancient Vedic scriptures speak of taking nothing without giving something back. Imagine what would happen if each time we took something, we gave something back. I don't think the Vedic writings were talking about trash. They were speaking to an inherent sense of reciprocity.

Stealing from the Future

We are not only stealing from the earth, we are stealing from the future and from our children and their children in such massive proportions it often feels like we are caught on a speeding train with no brakes and no way to get off. And yet we remain insatiable, a collective giant hole that we can't seem to fill. The excess in our bodies, our calendars, our closets, are all signs that we are living as if there is no tomorrow and no one to live here after we are gone.

We have lost our sense of gratitude. It is as if we had been invited to the most fabulous weekend at a friend's home where we enjoyed scrumptious meals and delightful entertainment only to leave without so much as a hint of a thank you. Our focus seems to be on what we don't have or what we might not have in the future, rather than on the abundance right before us.

If we stop long enough to gaze at what is laid out before us, to let the mystery of beauty and the wonder of the seasons sit deeply in our soul, our hearts cannot help but burst forth in thanksgiving and gratitude to life itself. Inborn to this kind of wonder is gratitude for where our life came from and indebtedness to the future. I am reminded of the native wisdom

अस्तेय

to make all decisions as if they mattered seven generations into the future.

I recently saw the play *Handing Down the Names* by Steven Dietz. It is the story of two hundred years of German ancestors, beginning with those who left the German states to become farmers along the Volga River in Russia, eventually immigrating to America. The story is profound in its ability to show the strength of a people and their love and hope for future generations. As Dietz states, "My ancestors picked sugar beets for generations so that now, in 1995, I can pick words. Tell stories."

I left the play with intense emotion. My ancestors sacrificed so much for me. They endured hardships beyond my comprehension with only one thought, that of the upcoming generations. They literally gave their lives to create beauty on the earth and better times for the future. In that moment, I realized the incredible love that my life stands on. Remembering our ancestors and the mystery that brought us into being is a way to reframe the sacredness of our own lives and the sacredness of the lives that will come after us. It is to find ourselves as current caretakers in this

From the standpoint of my teenage granddaughter and her friends, they are inheriting a huge mess that feels almost insurmountable.

lineage of past and future lives. It is to find ourselves with our direction pointed to those who will come after us.

I felt this lineage the other night when I was up into the early morning hours having a discussion with my teenage granddaughter. In this conversation she chose to express her view of what is facing her. From the standpoint of her and her friends, they are inheriting a huge mess that feels almost insurmountable. In chemistry class they had covered the capabilities of nuclear destruction, the long shelf life of nuclear material, and the challenge of nuclear disposal. In another class they spoke of the world's hatred and fear of this country. In another class they spoke of the challenges and choices they will have to make about genetic research. As she continued, I could only shake my head and say, "I'm so sorry; it shouldn't be this way for you." My heart felt heavy.

Stealing from Ourselves

Not only do we steal from others, the earth, and the future; we steal from our own lives. In all the ways that we impose an outside image of ourselves onto ourselves, we are stealing from the unfolding of our own uniqueness. All demands and expectations that we place on ourselves steal from our own enthusiasm. All self-sabotage, lack of belief in ourselves, low self-esteem, judgments, criticisms, and demands for perfection are forms of self-abuse in which we destroy the very essence of our vitality. All the ways we live in the past or future steal from ourselves. And all the ways we put up fences, whether real or imagined, around our physical belongings or around our mental idealisms, we put up barriers that steal from the full expansion of our own lives.

> We need to take time to rest and to reflect and to contemplate.

We are captured in a culture where our very identity is tied up with our accomplishments. We wear all we have to do like a badge on our shirt for all to see. In this rush to get to the next thing, we have left no time for ourselves to digest and assimilate our lives; this may be our biggest theft of all. We need time to catch up with ourselves. We need time to chew and ponder and allow the experiences of life to integrate within us. We need time to rest and to reflect and to contemplate.

I experienced the truth of this need a few years ago when I was on the fast track. After three years at a grueling pace, I woke up one morning to realize I no longer had access to the experience of my life. It was one of the strangest feelings I have ever had. I have no other words to describe the feeling except to say that I no longer could remember any experiences of where I had been or what I had done. It was just too much for my system. I was on overload and my system shut down. It just quit. I had taken no time in those three years for even the semblance of reflection or integration; it was just on to the next thing, full speed ahead. Because I had not taken time to pause and allow my experiences to become part of me, I did not get to keep the experiences, they were gone. I had stolen this part of my life from myself.

Shifting Our Focus

Small children, as they reach a certain age, begin to want what the other one has. It doesn't matter what it is, they want it. Looking at the state of the world, it seems many adults are still caught in the toddler stage of wanting what the other one has. The tenet of *Asteya*, or nonstealing, asks us to shift our focus from the other to ourselves. It asks us to get excited about the possibilities for our own life. When we attend to our own growth and learning in the area of our interests, we are engaged in the joy and challenge of building ourselves. From the fullness of our own talent and skill, we automatically serve the world rather than steal from it. This shifting of focus is illustrated by the following example.

> When we are engaged in the joy and challenge of building ourselves, we automatically serve the world rather than steal from it.

In India, during major festivities, elephants are paraded down the narrow streets, proudly dressed in silks and jewelry, carrying the likeness of a deity on their backs. Along the way, vendors, displaying luscious treats and sparkling jewelry, are numerous. The elephants, being curious and playful by nature, can't help but swing their trunks this way and that in an attempt to capture the glitter and treats lining the streets. Destruction and chaos quickly follow. However, the trainers, knowing their elephant's adventuresome nature, have learned to coax them into wrapping their trunks around a bamboo shoot. Now, as the elephants march down the street carrying their bamboo shoot, the parade continues smoothly.

We are much like those elephants. When we don't know what we want or we don't have the courage to pursue it, everything that everyone else is doing looks tempting to us. We begin to lust after others' accomplishments and others' possessions. We get sidetracked from our own dreams and our own realness. However, when we are focused on our own dreams, we can move forward with dignity, much like those elephants holding onto the bamboo shoot, undisturbed by the glitter and sparkle along the way. By holding on to our "bamboo shoot," we can begin to build our competency and create the circumstances within us to have what we want.

Building Our Competence

My spouse tells a story about how he used to glue himself to the TV to watch the Olympics every four years. There he would sit, slumped over in his chair, hour after hour, with mayonnaise on his protruding bare belly from eating more food than he needed, telling himself that when the next Olympic games rolled around, he would be representing the United States as a skilled, in shape, athlete. When the next Olympics rolled around, he was still in the chair watching, a spectator to what he wanted.

The Sanskrit word *adikara* means the right to know or the right to have. This word challenges us to the reality that if we want something, then we better grow the competency required to have it. Like the story above, we can dream and wish all we want, but we only get what we have the competency to have and keep. Anything else is stealing.

Think about people who win big bucks in the lottery and within a year are back to being broke. Or think of CEO's who run companies into the ground because they don't have the skill to manage a huge corporation. In both of these cases, these people are stealing; they are trying to have something beyond their competency. Our outcomes in life are consistent with our abilities, not necessarily our wishes or goals.

Competency includes the ability to see what is right before us. I used to tell myself the story that I worked hard and prayed hard, but never really got what I was after. Now, as I look back, I understand that I didn't have the competency to see that what I had worked for and asked for was right in front of me and I couldn't contain it or sometimes even see it!

A colander is an excellent example of *adikara*. We may seek something so earnestly and yet, if we are full of holes like the colander, what we want will always elude us. Building our *adikara* is plugging our holes by growing our competency in the area of our desires. Building our competency takes practice and learning.

Preparing ourselves to hold what we want is an exciting, full-time job. It moves us away from any victim stories into full responsibility for our lives. How many times do we wish for more money, but we wouldn't have a clue what to do with it (at least sensibly) if it did show up? *Asteya,* or nonstealing, demands that we become capable of stewarding what we ask for. Learn about money and investments, be savvy with the money you do have, be prepared, be generous; have the *adikara* for what you want.

You may have seen the delightful film *My Big Fat Greek Wedding.* Nia Vardalos was a struggling comedian who told stories about her Greek background and her non-Greek husband. Rita Wilson, wife of Tom Hanks, caught Nia's comedy routine one evening, loved it, and thought her story would make a great movie. Nia Vardalos was prepared. She had already written the movie script. In Nia's words, "Rita Wilson is Greek and she came to the show and she said this should be a movie and I handed her the screenplay. She sent her husband

अस्तेय

Tom Hanks to the show; he called me up and he said, 'We're going to make your movie and you're going to play the lead role.'" Nia Vardalos was ready.

If we are not prepared to contain our deep desires, we can easily find ourselves stealing in all kinds of inappropriate and destructive ways. This jewel asks us instead to focus on our desires and then build the competency to have them. It leaves us with the question, "Are you available to what you want?" It opens the door for us to seek out mentors and learn from people who have already accomplished what we are seeking; it also opens the door to the fun of learning new things. We can find someone more accomplished and skilled (maybe even radical) than we are and learn from them how to plug our own holes of incompetence. And so that we don't steal from them, we can compensate them fairly.

When I realized that somewhere along the line I had forgotten how to play, I hired my teenage granddaughter as my play coach. Not only did she enjoy creating scenarios for our playtime and giving me play assignments to do on my own (and getting paid as her grandma's coach), but the whole process brought me into a new world of adventure and fun, as well as deepening my relationship with my granddaughter.

In the book *The Ultimate Gift* by Jim Stovall, we meet a self-made billionaire named Red who is about to die. Discerning where to leave his companies, investments, and other assets, Red looks at his family and sees only selfishness and greed, a family spoiled by the money that has made their lives so easy. Red decides to make amends with his one grandson. The story unfolds as, after Red's death, the will is read to a family gathered in high expectation, only to leave one by one angry at what the will has revealed. However to grandson Jason, Red leaves twelve tasks that must be fulfilled in order for Jason to receive his inheritance of unknown monetary value. Task by task, a begrudging Jason learns important lessons about the value of work, friendship, service, etc. until he has become an entirely different person. Rather than a spoiled trust fund baby, Jason is now a competent, compassionate, skilled leader, ready to give millions away to people and projects that can make a difference. In case you aren't familiar with the story line, I won't spoil it for you. Suffice it to say, by the time we know what the full monetary value of Jason's inheritance is, it doesn't matter to Jason or to us.

In the story above, the grandfather had the foresight to give his grandson step-by-step tasks that, should he succeed at each task, would grow Jason into a person competent to have a billion dollars worth of investments handed to him. I think life is like this. It gives us tasks, that should we succeed, grow us into the kind of people that life can trust with important things. And, like Jason, often we mistake these tasks as a burden rather than an opportunity to grow our compassion and skill level. The grandfather knew that it is not the accumulation of things that ultimately gives us satisfaction, but the accumulation of values and competency. The jewel of nonstealing, asks us to build our competency with life itself.

Where stealing unleashes pain and suffering on our self and others, building our competency opens up a world of joy and possibility. It is a grand adventure to turn our attention away from stealing and towards the life long task of shaping ourselves into someone of value. ↩

अस्तेय

Questions for Exploration

Living with these questions, taking time for reflection, and journaling will give you new insights into your life and the practice of nonstealing. For this month, frame your exploration in the following statement by Albert Einstein:

*A hundred times a day
I remind myself
that my inner and outer life
depend on the labors of other people,
living and dead,
And that I must exert myself
in order to give
in the full measure I have received
and am still receiving.*

Week One: This week notice when and how you steal from others through time, attention, "one-upmanship," power, confidence, and not being able to celebrate others' successes. Notice what is happening in you that prompts this stealing. Now practice being a "forklift" so that everyone you come into contact with feels uplifted because they were in your presence.

Week Two: This week notice where you are stealing from the earth and stealing from the future. Where are you taking without returning something of at least equal value? This week, live in reciprocity with the earth and awareness of the future.

Week Three: This week live as a visitor to this world, rather than an owner. Notice how much is available to you to use and enjoy without needing to own them (parks, libraries, concerts, sunsets, etc.).

Week Four: This week think about your dreams and goals and make a list of things to do/study/try that would increase your knowledge and competency and bring you closer to your goal, thus building your *adikara*.

For this month ponder the words of Albert Einstein and live in gratitude and reciprocity with what you have been given. ℮

BRAHMACHARYA

In the dark and muck,
a golden lotus blossoms ~
God's grace awaits us.
~ C.L.

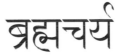

Brahmacharya: Nonexcess

There is a commercial I still remember vividly from my childhood years. In the commercial, a very miserable man has just gorged himself on too much food. Gripped in the pangs of lethargy, gas, and bloating, he miserably proclaims, "I can't believe I ate the whole thing." Perhaps I remember this commercial because of the times I, too, have found myself in the lingering after effects of overindulgence. I know firsthand the misery of a too full stomach, the deadness of overwork, the lethargy of oversleep. As I sit in the heaviness of excess, I find myself once again in disbelief that I have done this to myself, and hear myself utter words similar to the above, "I can't believe I ate the whole thing." And all I can do is suffer and watch how the overindulgence has imposed itself on the joy of the moment.

Whether we find ourselves overdoing food, work, exercise, or sleep, excess is often a result of forgetting the sacredness of life. The fourth jewel, *Brahmacharya*, literally means "walking with God" and invites us into an awareness of the sacredness of all of life. This guideline is a call to leave greed and excess behind and walk in this world with wonder and awe, practicing nonexcess and attending to each moment as holy.

Brahmacharya has been interpreted by many to mean celibacy or abstinence. Although this could certainly be one form that *Brahmacharya* takes, its implications are much more broad. It does, however, imply dealing with the passion of our sexuality, as well as our other desires, in a manner that is sacred and life-giving, rather than excessive.

On a recent trip to India, I met a man named Thakur who was the first man to bring trekking and other outdoor adventures to that part of the Himalayas. He was a successful business man, living the long hours and impositions of success. He told me, however, that wealthy as he was, he still lived in the home his father had built on the outskirts of the village. The door to this home was chest high, so entering the home required him to bow his head. He said this simple action of bowing as he entered, reminded him of the sacredness of all things and he spent his evenings and his sleep in peace and ease, ready to bring that same sacredness to his business negotiations the next day.

> *Brahmacharya* reminds us to enter each day and each action with a sense of holiness rather than indulgence.

Brahmacharya is like this low entrance for us, it reminds us to enter each day and each action with a sense of holiness rather than indulgence, so that our days may be lived in the wonder of sacredness rather than the misery of excess.

Nonexcess ~ Taming Our Overindulgence

The number of sheds and storage units, the attractive plastic storage bins that fill rows in our stores, the statistics on American obesity, and the shortage of waste facilities for our trash are all neon signs that we are a people of excess. We overdo sex, we overdo food, we overdo work, we overdo sleep, we overdo entertainment, we overdo our material possessions, and often we overdo our spirituality. We seem far from grasping the concept of "enough."

In yogic thought, there is a moment in time when we reach the perfect limit of what we are engaged in. If we take food for instance, we gain energy and vitality from the food we are eating – up to a point. If we continue to eat past that point, there is a downward turn into lethargy. If we eat slowly enough and pay attention, we can find this point that sits perfectly on the line of "just right." It is this moment of "just enough" that we need to recognize. Past that point, we begin our descent into excess. This same process is true for any activity that we are engaged in.

> In yogic thought, there is a moment in time when we reach the perfect limit of what we are engaged in. It is this moment of "just enough" that we need to recognize.

I watched my granddaughter Aryka practice this place of "just enough." She had asked for some scrambled eggs, so I made her a scrambled egg the way she likes it. She demolished it hungrily with comments of how delicious it was. Then she asked for more. I made her a second egg and the scenario was repeated. When she asked for a third egg, which I obliged, she began to eat it with comments of contentment. Midway through her third bite, she exclaimed, "Grandma, this egg tastes terrible, something is wrong with it." I marveled that she could pay such close attention to know that what had been so satisfying to her was now distasteful because she had had enough.

Why do we move past the place of enough into excess? Yogic thought tells us it is because our mind begins to connect certain emotional states with certain foods or activities. There is a difference between say, the body's need to satisfy thirst and the extravagant things the mind does with this simple desire. A desire that could easily be fulfilled with a glass of water somehow, in our mind's convoluted way, gets hooked up with memories and conditioning tied to emotional satisfaction or emotional disturbance. When a certain emotional attachment is placed with a simple body need, we can find ourselves in trouble. Without realizing it, we have acquired an addiction-like need for the repetition of the feelings associated with that thing.

Why do we move past the place of enough into excess?

My business partner, Ann, and I went through a phase where we were drinking chai almost daily. We were working hard and having fun together, and the chai became both a reward and a treat for us. Our need was to satisfy our thirst, but the memory that began to take hold of both of us was that we needed the chai to satisfy us. And, with each chai, we expected to feel the same pleasure of companionship and the satisfaction of work well done. There is nothing wrong with drinking chai, in fact it is quite enjoyable, but we soon realized that we weren't having the chai, the chai was having us. Now we had an addiction, not the simple need to satisfy thirst. Our minds had created the need for the feeling of reward, not to simply enjoy the pleasure of a chai.

As we begin to peel ourselves out of our web of excess, it is important to check in with the body's needs and to get skilled at separating these bodily needs from the mind's stories. Sometimes the need is to feel sadness. When this feeling comes upon us, the mind may trick us into thinking we need to do something or to eat something. I found this experience to be true for me when my mother died. While my mother was alive, one of our favorite things to do together was to stay up late into the night watching a movie and eating ice cream. After her death, I found myself "craving" late night movies and ice cream. When I checked in with my body, it was clear that I was tired and full. In truth, I was missing my mom and I needed to face the grief. To indulge in a movie and ice cream would have left me with excess weariness in my body and excess food in my stomach. And I would still be missing my mom. I needed to separate my mind's story from my body's needs and simply let myself cry.

We are here on this world, in part, to feel enjoyment and pleasure. If we are in the pleasure and not the addiction, we are practicing *Brahmacharya*. If we are feeding our mental stories and have moved past bodily comfort, we are in addiction and out of harmony with this guideline. Nonexcess is not about nonenjoyment. It actually is about enjoyment and pleasure in its fullest experience. The questions before us are: Are you eating the food, or is the food eating you? Are you doing the activity, or is the activity doing you? Can you enjoy pleasure without excess? In answering these questions, we have to be able to discern between what the body needs

> We have to be able to discern between what the body needs in the moment and the story our mind is telling us.

in the moment and the story our mind is telling us. (I don't know about you, but I have personally noticed that sugar, salt, and caffeine create more mind stories than lettuce does!) We also must be fearless in facing our sadness, grief, and disappointments without needing to soothe them with food or sex.

When I was in Nicaragua, I was able to hear the Minister of the Interior speak about the state of affairs in his country. At that time there was a large contingent of people from the United States bringing their faith to the people of Nicaragua. Part of their evangelizing was the sharing of large tables of exotically prepared food at their gatherings. The Minister of Interior, choosing to not attend these affairs, was quick to comment on the food in this way, "When the organisms in my tummy are over happy, I can't think straight." Overindulgence snuffs out the life force like too many logs on a fire overpowers the fire. Practicing nonexcess preserves and honors this life force within us, so that we can live with clarity and sacredness.

If we find ourselves living in the extremes of addiction, excess, and overindulgence in any place in our life, then fasting, celibacy, or abstinence can be very useful to bring us back to the fullness of pleasure. Fasting and celibacy are both strong practices to pull in the reins, find our center, and take stock of our lives. Going through times in our lives when abstinence or fasting is imposed on us, either through our own or our partner's illness, can be times of great cleansing for us and lead to greater discernment of our tendencies towards excess and the stories the mind has made up about these tendencies.

Walking with God

Brahmacharya invites us to live with God, not excess. This guideline invites us into the sanctity of all life by seeing every relationship we have as a relationship with the Divine and by seeing every experience we have as an experience of the Divine. Can you honor all as sacred? Can you honor yourself as sacred? If we stop and pause for a moment, we know that it is the simple things that stir our soul and bless us with happiness. The wind in the trees, the colors of the sky, the touch of a loved one, the delight of a child, a shared moment with a friend, can fill us to overflowing. This overflowing is expansive and humbling, much different than the satiation of excess.

> Can you honor all as sacred? Can you honor yourself as sacred?

If we stop and reflect on our lives or out at the world, we can see an innate intelligence about things. It is as if a beautiful tapestry is being woven and we are one of the colors of thread being moved by a needle held by something greater than we are. It is this greatness, the Master Weaver, which we seek to be in touch with. When we see with the eyes of mystery, we begin to see the sacred in the ordinary and the ordinary in the sacred. Every task becomes an opportunity to wonder and be amazed. Mending the split between what we see as important or not, and who we see as important or not, puts us on the path to cherishing all people and all tasks. Media, culture, even our own egos separate, divide and then rank. We are asked to bring it all together and cherish it all by seeing the thread of the divine at play.

Seeing with the eyes of holiness shifts how we act as well as how we see. There is an inbuilt need to pause and give thanks. There is an inbuilt need to open the heart in wonder. When gratitude and wonder sit in the heart, there is no need for excess. Seeing everything as holy brings a continuity to life; it grounds us in centeredness. Whereas excess overdoes us, overextends us, and takes us away from ourselves, seeing everything as sacred firmly roots us and balances us.

I have found that when the sense of wonder leaves me, when everything becomes dull and ordinary, it is because I have kept too fast a pace for too long. I have pushed past my own boundaries and now I am out of balance. It is time to rest. When I am rested, nothing is dull and ordinary; everything glows with mystery. Whether I take it easy for a day or escape into the woods by myself, it is hard to give this rest to myself. There are a million and one reasons why I can't. My ego likes to feel important, and it doesn't feel very important when I am resting. My ego also doesn't like the idea that

> Seeing with the eyes of holiness shifts how we act as well as how we see. When gratitude and wonder sit in the heart, there is no need for excess.

life can go on without me, even if it is only for a few hours; I like to be where the action is. Besides, in this culture of constant activity, there is always so much that needs to be done.

And yet I am hungry to step outside of the habits of technology and the bombardment of stimulation and the routines I have conveniently put in place for myself. I am hungry to learn from the silence and see if I am on track with my soul. I am hungry to tame the stimulation and pull back the indulgences. And I am hungry to do nothing and let that be more than enough. Resting rejuvenates my sense of mystery. In this simple act, I find my eyes are shifted to wonder and my heart spontaneously bursts with songs of gratitude.

The Divine is so magnificent, weaving a design of intricacy and mastery in an extravagance beyond our understanding. Such magnificence deserves an audience to marvel and appreciate it. I think following this jewel is like being an audience for God and may mean shifting our days so we have more time to just watch and marvel. It may mean adding more ritual to our lives and a certain rhythm. We may shift some of our commitments so that we have the time to see and attend to mystery and holiness by lighting candles, saying prayers, massaging our feet, taking hikes, or rubbing our loved one's back.

Being an audience of the divine mystery begins to shift us out of clock time and into a divine rhythm. I had this experience of shifting rhythm when I took a solo one month Sabbatical to a lakeside cabin. Somewhere in that month, I got captured. Without a clock dictating my next step or my usual habits manipulating the moment, I got swept up by a universal rhythm that I came to call "God's heartbeat." I hiked and kayaked, ate and slept, read and wrote, and did my practice, but these weren't separate activities or accomplishments, they were more like rhythm. I was a cell in the heart of God and the beating of God's heart moved me. The doings and nondoings wove together in one harmonious rhythm.

In that month I learned that the rhythm of mystery

looks nothing like the demands of clock time. God's time isn't logical to our limited minds; it doesn't plan and it doesn't keep track, but somehow the dishes still got done and the meals cooked. It just happened from a different place. When I didn't know the day, or the time, or the temperature, an innate intelligence began to set the next thing in motion. I moved without moving and all I saw was beauty and wonder. Without a schedule or a plan, being and doing blended until they felt the same. There was no purpose, except for the pure delight of the moment. God's heartbeat.

> As we move deeper into the practice of "walking with God," we will find that excess doesn't own us quite as much as it used to.

When I returned from my month, I found myself once again with a watch on my wrist, a cell phone in my hand, and my computer on standby. And I found myself face to face with the accusation of Vimalananda who stated, "In this country, you wear your God on your wrist." This guideline of *Brahmacharya* asks us if we can use these objects of technology as guides to help us maneuver through society's demands and expectations without them becoming gods. Can we instead move to the rhythm of the universe as a cell in the heart of mystery?

I have read many self help books and have benefited greatly from them. That said, I think mystery is what begins to shape-shift us into a deeper understanding of our humanity. As we move deeper into the practice of "walking with God," we will find that excess doesn't own us quite as much as it used to.

When we get the real nourishment that divine mystery gives us, the pretend nourishment of excess becomes less and less interesting to us.

Being an audience for God also means we have to get off center stage. We don't need to be the center of attention and activity all the time. I think it might surprise us to realize how much crazy activity we create in our days just so we can feel important. We wear our busyness like a badge, like our busyness would somehow impress the rest of the world, or impress ourselves. How many of us go to bed with a sense of accomplishment because we checked a lot of things off our task list or someone told

> Howard Thurman said, "Don't ask yourself what the world needs. Ask yourself what makes you come alive."

us how "great" we were, or we "helped" others? What if walked off stage altogether and put God there instead. Maybe then we could go to sleep at night, not with a sense of accomplishment, but with a sense of wonder, because all day we had been an attentive audience to the divine play.

Brahmacharya reminds us that we aren't embodied in this form to feel dead but to feel alive. We aren't embodied to snuff out our vitality and passion through excess but to bring it to full expression. *Brahmacharya* invites us to be willing to walk around "turned on" to the wonders of life itself. Howard Thurman understood the importance of our passion to the world when he said, "Don't ask yourself what the world needs. Ask yourself what makes you come alive. And then go do it. Because what the world needs is people who have come alive." ⋸〉

ब्रह्मचर्य

Questions for Exploration

Living with these questions, taking time for reflection, and journaling will give you new insights into your life and the practice of nonexcess. For this month, frame your exploration in the following statement by Joseph Campbell:

> Be true to the purpose and limits
> of each thing in existence.
> Behave purely and serve purely
> the reality of what you are given
> by making every human function
> without exception
> a religious act
> of sacrifice and worship.

Week One: This week examine your beliefs, values, habits, and actions around sexuality and sexual activity. Notice what your culture, the media, your faith community, and your family have to say about this topic. Then notice if you act on outside authority, or your own beliefs.

Week Two: This week live in nonexcess. Eat, work, and sleep to the point of increased energy and before the lethargy of excess sets in. Ponder the words of Gensei, a Japanese Buddhist monk, who said, "The point in life is to know what's enough." For this week, know what is enough and stop there. Practice pleasure without excess.

Week Three: This week notice where you see God and where you don't. Notice the beliefs or judgments that limit your ability to see God and experience God in all things. Then practice letting everything be a relationship with the Divine. See the sacred in the ordinary and God in each person you encounter. Ponder the words of Yogi Bhajan, "If you can't see God in all, you can't see God at all." See God in all.

Week Four: This week contemplate your own divinity. Are you willing to be sacred? Write down three practices that connect you to your passion and your sacredness.

For this month ponder the words of Joseph Campbell and live the sacredness of your life. ⁛

APARIGRAHA

Fall deeply in love.
Cherish all in your heart. Now
open and let go!
~ C.L.

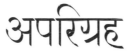

Aparigraha: Nonpossessiveness

I remember when my children were small and I would pick them up at child care. It didn't matter how much fun they were having with yummy treats to eat or new toys to explore or new friends to play with. The minute I entered the room, they dropped everything and ran as fast as they could into my waiting arms. Nothing was more important to them than I was. As they grew older, however, the toys became more and more interesting to them, until at times, I would show up and they would totally ignore me.

Much like small children, we live in a world with an abundance of treats and toys and friends. They are there for us to enjoy, but never in place of the one who gives these gifts. The jewel of *Aparigraha* invites us to enjoy life to the fullest and yet always be able to drop everything and run into the waiting arms of the Divine. If we prefer to play with our toys, we have missed the point.

Aparigraha, or nonpossessiveness, can also be interpreted as nonattachment, nongreed, nonclinging, nongrasping, and noncoveting; we can simply think of it as being able to "let go." The sadhus of India recognize how easy it is to become attached to things of this world. Sadhus don the color orange and take vows to renounce all worldly pleasures in favor of the Divine. They spend most of their time in the forests, away from any temptations that might become more interesting to them than their companionship with Divinity. Although this is an extreme example, it shows one way of staying free of the prison of possessiveness.

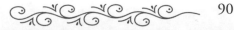

For those of us who choose to stay immersed in the world, loving and living fully without becoming attached is not an easy thing. When we experience the completeness of being loved, the satisfaction of a superb meal, the acknowledgment of work well done, we can easily want to hold on to these moments and never let them go. It is easy to want the same satisfaction and begin to demand the same fulfillment from these things again and again. But it is the nature of things to change and by failing to let them change or move on, they begin to disappoint us and our attempts to hold on begin to make us stale and discontent. What we try to possess, possesses us.

> *Aparigraha* invites us to let go and to pack lightly for our journey through life, all the while caring deeply and enjoying fully.

How do we move through life loving deeply and engaging fully without getting attached? Looking at the inhalation and exhalation of the breath, the timing of trapeze artists, and an ancient practice of catching monkeys can give us glimpses into the ability to let go rather than be attached. The guideline of *Aparigraha* invites us to let go and to pack lightly for our journey through life, all the while caring deeply and enjoying fully.

The Breath as Teacher

What if we could trust life like we trust the breath? What if we could take in all the nourishment of the moment and then let it go fully, trusting that more nourishment will come?

Just like the breath gives us nourishment, so does life in the form of homes, work, relationships, routines that bring ease, beliefs, stances, and images of ourselves. There is nourishment until we get attached to these things, often unconsciously, and then disturb ourselves with expectations, opinions, criticisms, disappointments, all because we forget to trust life, exhale, and let go. Like the breath when it is held too long, the things that nourish us can become toxic.

Aparigraha invites us to practice divine play, experience full intimacy and contact with the moment, and then to let go so the next thing can come. It is how our *adikara,* or competency, grows and how we become more who we are capable of becoming. I have a grand piano that I enjoy playing. But, as Yogiraj Achala reminds me, when it is time to eat I don't carry the piano to the dining room. Why would I want all that weight on my shoulders?

And yet, often we do try to carry the piano to the dining room table, so to speak, trying all different ways we can think of to find some kind of permanence, something to hold on to. But the nature of the realm of *Aparigraha* is impermanence. Everything changes. Nothing stays the same. If we can fall back to the breath and watch the belly rise and fall with each inhalation and exhalation, we can feel the truth of the transience of all things.

Hanging in Mid-Air

Much like the moment when the breath is completely exhaled, the trapeze artist has a moment when they are suspended in mid-air. My understanding is that they have to let go of one bar and wait in mid-air for the next swinging bar to reach them. If they hold on to the current bar, or reach for the next bar, their timing will be off and they will fall. Instead, they must let go fully to be ready for the bar swinging towards them, trusting the timing of the swing and not their own effort to reach.

> Like the breath when it is held too long, the things that nourish us can become toxic.

I'm not a trapeze artist, but my experience of letting go feels very much like being suspended in mid-air with nothing to hold on to. It is raw, naked, vulnerable, and uncomfortable. I would much prefer to let go when I know for sure what is coming. And when I have let go, I want to somehow stay connected, just in case I want it back. To let go completely feels like a suspension in the void.

The practice of nonclinging is as free as swinging from bar to bar effortlessly, in perfect trust and perfect timing. Any kind of holding too long or grasping too far forward in an effort to maintain a sense of security is deadly to our spiritual growth and the natural unfolding of our lives.

Let Go of the Banana!

I am fascinated by an ancient process of capturing monkeys in India. Like the breath and the trapeze artist, this process gives us insights into how we stay attached to objects of life and how deadly that can become. In this process of catching monkeys, small cages with narrow bars are made and a banana is placed inside the cage. The monkeys come along, reach in between the bars, and grab the banana. Then the monkeys begin the impossible task of trying to pull the banana through the bars. And here is the amazing thing – in the moment when the monkey catchers come along, the monkeys are totally free. There is nothing keeping them from running off to safety as they hear danger approach. All they have to do is to let go of the banana. Instead, they refuse to release the banana and are easily taken into captivity.

"Bananas" for us are anything we expect to give us the same fulfillment the second and third time. When we expect our spouse to make us feel good like they did the evening before, or when we expect a dinner out to satisfy us like it did the last time, or when we expect to be appreciated like we were yesterday, indeed anytime we want the same "feel good" results, we are "holding on to the banana." Our expectations keep us captive and often disgruntled.

> Our expectations keep us captive and often disgruntled, and yet we choose our attachments rather than our freedom.

The image of the monkey holding on to the banana is real for those of us captured in our attachments. Indeed, nothing is holding us. We, like the monkeys, are totally free. Instead, we choose to hold on, choosing our attachments and our greed rather than our freedom. To choose freedom, we simply need to "let go of the banana." Instead, we create our own prison of captivity. What we hold, begins to hold us. As illustrated in the following example, captivity can also be an image of our self that we insist on holding.

अपरिग्रह

What we Possess, Possesses Us

When I went through a tough divorce with two small children, I decided then and there that I would never need anyone again. Unconsciously, that decision began to work on me in ways I didn't recognize: I would refuse to ask for help or to accept help when it was offered; I refused to let myself be tired or to rest; I refused to be anything but invincible. I was never going to find myself that vulnerable again.

It was decades later that I began to realize the havoc that my attachment to this image of myself was having on my life. I was wearing myself out and wearing out everyone around me. I couldn't stop because if I stopped, I might feel that sense of helplessness again. I was holding on to an image that was in turn holding on to me and keeping me in bondage. The play and spontaneity and fun in my life were becoming almost nonexistent. Invincibility was eating all the joy out of my life.

Anything we cling to creates a maintenance problem for us. The material items that we hoard, collect, buy because they are on sale or take because they are "free," all take up space and demand our attention. Storage boxes and sheds become an easy way to fool ourselves. Subtle attachments come in the form of our images and beliefs about ourselves, about how life should be, about how others should be. These images keep us in bondage to our own learning and growth. Clutter in our physical space blocks our ability to physically move, while

> Anything we cling to creates a maintenance problem for us.

clutter in our minds blocks our freedom to expand and have space for the next thing life wants to bring to us.

I went through a period of attachment to bean and rice burritos made at our local co-op deli. It didn't matter who was behind the counter, they all knew me and they knew exactly what I wanted, even the special request for extra filling. On one visit, the server behind the deli began to fix my burrito and made the comment, "You are so boring." Another time when I was particularly craving my usual, I stopped at the deli in full anticipation of the upcoming indulgence, only to find out they were all out of bean and rice mix for burritos. I was irate and devastated. In that moment I witnessed the severity of my attachment when I was unwilling to substitute another kind of burrito, instead choosing to have my day ruined.

What I was holding onto was holding on to me. Attachments ruin our day when they aren't fulfilled. Attachments make us boring. And attachments keep us blinded to the smorgasbord of new opportunities around us.

The word attachment can be traced to a root word that means "to nail." Attachments are like nailing ourselves to our need for someone or something to continue to be the same and to always be there for us in the same way. When we nail ourselves to our needs for others, to our feelings, our roles, our agendas, our pleasures, our identities, we become more like rats in a maze than free human beings.

Just how Many Bags are you Taking?

Recently my teenage granddaughter and I went on our first overnight retreat adventure together. In my usual organized, prepared style, I started asking her way in advance what we should pack. I held my frustration as the days passed and the question continued to go unanswered. The day before we were to leave, I said, "Ashly, we have to make plans." "Grandma," she said, "that's the whole point of getting away; make it easy, don't take anything, not even plans." Further conversation revealed her packing list: a book, a soccer ball, and a healthy supply of her favorite organic frozen dinners.

I found myself stunned at the simplicity of her understanding of retreat time. In my mind I reviewed the large amounts of packing and preparation that had always burdened my retreat time. Excited at the opportunity, I leaped into this new challenge before me to "take nothing with me." I would like to report that my efforts were a success, but alas, the morning we left found us both filling the car with all kinds of last minute baggage.

But the seed had been planted in my mind and I found myself wondering where else I was "missing the point" with my planning and packing and hauling. In fact, how many suitcases full of expectations, tasks, plans, resentments, and unforgiven moments was I toting around with me every day? Even airlines know to charge a fine when we pack over the limit I thought to myself, and yet I wonder how many of us are packing over the limit every morning and wearying ourselves throughout the day with this heavy baggage?

> How many suitcases full of expectations, tasks, plans, resentments, and unforgiven moments was I toting around with me every day?

What if we woke up every morning and took nothing with us? What if that was the whole point? What if we unpacked our way to God? Unpacked our way to freedom? Unpacked our way to being?

And yet, we seem to put more into our already full suitcases as the day wears on and we add some disappointments and maybe a little anger mixed with some frustration to our already heavy load. This craziness we do to ourselves is as silly as if we carried a heavy load of bricks around all day and continued to add more to our pile.

Pack light for the journey, my granddaughter reminded me. Strip yourself to raw nakedness and vulnerability, the yogis teach us. This is the invitation of nonpossessiveness. Are we up to the unpacking?

But Aren't we Supposed to Care?

Nonattachment does not mean that we don't care or that we somehow shut ourselves off from the pleasures and joy of life and each other. In fact, nonattachment frees us up to be immersed in appreciation of life and one another. We are asked to let go of the *clinging* to the thing, not the enjoyment of the thing itself. Letting go of the ownership opens us up to full engagement with what is set before us in the present moment. Life becomes a banquet, and

> Nonattachment does not mean that we don't care. In fact, nonattachment frees us up to be immersed in appreciation of life and one another.

we are free to feast. Like the breath, we are invited to breathe in deeply, enjoying the fullness of the inhalation, and then to let go just as deeply and fully, enjoying the release of the exhale.

The fewer attachments we carry with us, the more we are free to enjoy and engage and live every moment before us to the fullest. The more breath we let go of, the more room there is in our body for the fullness of the next inhalation. The more

> A bird cannot hold its perch and fly. Neither can we grasp anything and be free.

we generously share and give away, the more expansive and light we become. The journey of life is towards freedom. A bird cannot hold its perch and fly. Neither can we grasp anything and be free.

Practicing constant generosity and unfailing trust will keep our greed in check and keep us open to life's unfolding. What wants to come to us is so great. And what we hold on to is often so small. Like the trapeze artist, are we willing to be suspended in mid-air in total trust of the timing and of a future that is greater than the one we are holding on to? ✌

 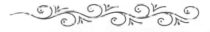

Questions for Exploration

Living with these questions, taking time for reflection, and journaling will give you new insights into your life and the practice of nonpossessiveness. For this month, frame your exploration in the following statement by Swami Jnaneshvara:

Love is what is left when
You've let go of
All the things you love.

Week One: This week pay attention to your breath. Let the simple act of inhaling and exhaling teach you about the fullness of breathing in life without the need to hold on to it. Journal your observations and experience.

Week Two: This week look at the physical things you have surrounded yourself with. Do these things make you feel free and light or do they have a hold on you and make you feel heavy? (Remember: what you cling to, clings to you.) Experience the difference between enjoyment and attachment.

Week Three: This week notice where you impose your expectations on people and things, unconsciously demanding that they give you the usual fulfillment and comfort. How do your expectations keep you limited and often disgruntled?

Week Four: Krishna Das makes the observation that in our country we have a muscle in the mind that we forget is there.

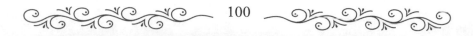

He calls it the "letting go" muscle. Krishna Das says we have developed a strong "holding on" muscle in the mind, but the "letting go" muscle is undeveloped. He suggests we get our mind in shape by using this muscle more often, practicing with little things so we are prepared when the bigger things come along. This week notice when you cling to experiences, emotions, thoughts, habits, and beliefs. Then give your "letting go" muscle some exercise and begin to let go.

For this month ponder the words of Swami Jnaneshvara and live fully in the experience of life without the burden of attachments or the need to possess. ᘒ

Reviewing the Yamas

Not long ago I was traveling with a friend who had just purchased a new Prius with a GPS (global positioning system). I enjoyed the adventure of having a computer talk to me and make sure I was on the right path. I laughed hilariously when my friend continued to drive straight after the computer had given instructions to turn right. The computer immediately responded with, "Drive forward and make an immediate legal U-turn."

The *Yamas* are like our personal GPS. They tell us when we are going in the wrong direction and that we need to make "an immediate legal U-turn." They let us know when we are making a negative impact on the world and invite us to "turn around" and take a step towards harmony instead.

The *Yamas* are not pat, simple answers; they are instructions to move in a certain direction. They require familiarity and daily practice. As our personal GPS, the practice of Nonviolence, Truthfulness, Nonstealing, Nonexcess, and Nonpossessiveness turn us:

- From harming ourselves and others to kindness and compassion for self and others
- From lies and half-truths to expressing our uniqueness and authenticity
- From theft to cultivating new skills and abilities
- From greed to appreciation and pleasure without excess
- From attachment to intimacy without possession

यम

The *Yamas* address the fact that we are social creatures, alive on a planet full of other life forms where we need to learn to live together and share the goods. The *Yamas*, or restraints, invite us into an adult relationship with the world, where we can see past our own needs into the collective good. In that sense, we can think of them as social disciplines, guiding us into harmony, peace, and right relationship with the world. The *Yamas* pull us back from needing so much that is external, and point us towards the unique expression of our own life. It is here that we feel the excitement and joy of living.

As we turn now to the disciplines of the *Niyamas*, we move our attention from an adult relationship with the world to an adult relationship with ourselves; and from a social focus to an internal focus. ☙

Nonviolence	Turns us from harming self and others to kindness and compassion for self and others.
Truthfulness	Turns us from lies and half-truths to expressing our uniqueness and authenticity.
Nonstealing	Turns us from theft to cultivating new skills and abilities.
Nonexcess	Turns us from greed to appreciation and pleasure without excess.
Nonpossessiveness	Turns us from attachment to intimacy without possession.

SAUCHA

It was glistening
on the green Lady's Mantle ~
Dew so clear and pure.
~ C.L.

शौच

Saucha: Purity

In *The Ragamuffin Gospel,* Brennan Manning tells the story of a tense moment in a recovery room. A young female patient is lying in bed. Standing beside her is the surgeon who has just removed a tumor from the young woman's face. Her husband, also in the room, stands at a distance. The patient is looking at herself in a handheld mirror for the first time after the surgery. Staring at the obvious downward turned corner of one side of her mouth, she asks the surgeon if she will always look lopsided. The surgeon replies a solemn yes, noting that he had to cut a nerve to get the tumor out. In that crucial moment, where the silence betrays a young woman doubting her future physical appeal, the husband acts. He walks over to his wife and tells her that he thinks she looks kind of cute with one side of her mouth turned down. Then he looks at her tenderly, shapes his mouth like hers, matching lips to lips, and kisses her.

The jewel of *Saucha,* or purity, carries a two-fold meaning. First, *Saucha* invites us to purify our bodies, our thoughts, and our words. As we purify ourselves physically and mentally, we become less cluttered and heavy; purification brings about a brightness and clarity to our essence. Second, this guideline has a relational quality. No one in the above story could have known ahead of time what the outcome of the surgery would be. Yet in that moment, when the wife doubted her own appeal, the husband

> *Saucha* invites us to purify our bodies, our thoughts, and our words.

was able to be with her purely, and in that purity, support her sense of self and the beauty of their relationship.

These two practices of purity are interrelated. As we purify ourselves from the heaviness and clutter of toxins, distractions, and scatteredness, we gain clarity to meet each moment with integrity and freshness. We become more pure in our relationship with each moment.

Purity as a Cleansing Process

The yogis have many practices to purify their bodies. Some may make us react with a "no way, not in my lifetime" attitude. (Like running string through the nasal passages and out the mouth or running thirty-two yards of cotton strip through the digestive system, to name a few.) Other purifying processes may be easier for us to engage in or at least try, like the neti pot.* Breath practices and postures are means of purifying the body, as are meditating and following an ethical system, like the *Yamas* and *Niyamas*. We can say what we want about these practices, but one thing is clear: the yogis place a high priority on purification. Why this importance?

There is a great energy that lies, mostly dormant, within each of us. This is the energy of consciousness or awakening. We have all, at times, felt the movement of this energy: moments when tears silently well in our eyes with the stirring of overwhelming love; moments when beauty stops us and captures us in wonder; moments when contentment and well-being ooze from our pores; moments when the life force pulses through us like electricity making us vibrant and young;

---

*A neti pot is a container used to run salt water through the nostrils.

moments when deep wisdom bathes light on our unknowing; moments when awareness comes to us in technicolor. These are small tastes of what happens as the energy within us awakens.

To practice the guideline of purity is to engage in cleansing processes, both physical and mental, that prepare us for these kinds of experiences all the time. Cleansing strengthens the body and insulates the mind, preparing us for the awakening of the energy within us. Cleansing prepares us for the greatness of our spirit. Cleansing lightens us to experience more of the divine mystery.

Taking steps to cleanse and purify ourselves will look different for each of us. Cleansing doesn't have to be earth shattering or weird to begin to work its magic. It might take the form of increased physical exercise, or increased water intake, a day of fasting on fruit and juice, or perhaps a day of cleaning out closets. Maybe we will choose to spend a day purifying our tongue so that we speak nothing of harm or untruth for the entire day. Whatever form purifying takes, it always begins with an intention to "lighten" the load we are carrying.

Where are these "loads" for you? Maybe your body is carrying poisonous toxins from a poor diet. Maybe your mind is carrying the heavy baggage of victimhood or unforgiveness. Maybe your home and workspace are full of clutter and junk. All of these "loads" weigh down your body, mind, and spirit. They are real and they are heavy. The guideline of purity invites us to move into ease, to do what it takes to get rid of this heaviness, wherever we find it in our lives. Clean your body; clean your mind; clean your living and work space.

I am one who believes strongly in the power of confession and forgiveness. I have found that some of the things I carry from my past actions need to be confessed, sometimes to a trusted friend and sometimes to a piece of paper that is then ritually burned. For me, this is a necessary cleansing practice for past errors in judgment and selfishness. In any way that we hold on to past wounds, we injure ourselves and keep ourselves from the ability to be pure with what is current in our lives. Forgiveness of self and other is the most generous gift we can give ourselves.

Several years ago when I did my Kundalini yoga teacher training under Yogi Bhajan, I had the opportunity to have a private session with him and ask him anything I wanted. At that time he had given me the spiritual name *Amrit Dev,* meaning the sweet nectar and wisdom of the guru is within you. The question I chose to ask him was how to live into the fullness of my spiritual name. He began to laugh boisterously and with a twinkle in his eye and a strong Indian accent, he replied, "Your poop must smell like nectar and your pee must smell like nectar." He continued to chuckle loudly, and that was the end of my time with him.

> Whatever form purifying takes, it is always begins with an intention to "lighten" the load we are carrying.

I had to pick my jaw up off the floor before I could begin to contemplate what he had said. I now understand he was speaking directly to the idea of purity. That I should strive to live in such a way that everything that goes into me and everything that comes out of me is pure.

Yogi Bhajan's explanation of my name helped me begin to understand the difference between purification and cleanliness. Recently back from India, I am once again sorting through this difference. I spent almost two weeks in an ashram doing purification practices, but it took me two hours when I got home to be "American clean." In this country we almost obsess about cleanliness, but pay little attention to purity. Cleanliness is a process of scrubbing the outside of us; it changes our outer appearance. Purification works on our insides and changes our very essence. Although cleanliness is important, *Saucha* calls us to the inward journey of purification not the external appearance of cleanliness.

Purity as Relational

Saucha has a relational quality that asks us not only to seek purity in ourselves, but to seek purity with each moment by allowing it to be as it is. We are asked to be with life, with others, with things, with the day, with work, with the weather, as they are in the moment, not as we wish they were or think they should be or expect them to be. We fail this guideline in any of our attempts to change, judge, criticize, alter, control, manipulate, pretend, be disappointed, or check out. Purity is not our attempt to make something different than it is; rather it is to be pure in our relationship with it, as it is in the moment.

The difference between being pure *with* something

rather than trying to *make* something pure is a subtle and tricky distinction. We can easily find ourselves in an arrogant position, sitting on our high horse thinking we are bringing something better to the moment, or perhaps thinking that the moment isn't worth our attention, or maybe even finding ourselves feeling that the moment owes us something. When our thoughts or actions are presumptive like this we actually stain the purity of the moment. We are not to bring our idea of purity to the moment; we are simply to be with the moment as it is.

> The difference between being pure *with* something rather than trying to *make* something pure is a subtle and tricky distinction.

In order to be pure with something, we are asked to do a lot of subtraction. We have to subtract all of our ideals, illusions, and expectations of "what should be" and "how we want it to be." We even have to drop our image of purity itself to begin to live in the oasis of this jewel. When we find ourselves stuck in a traffic jam, disappointed with our meal, tripping over messes in the house, or dealing with a crabby family member, we are invited to simply be with these times in a pure way, not to judge them as impure moments.

My sister-in-law recently returned from visiting her two-year-old grandson. She was fresh and alive from the experience. All she could talk about was how everything looked new to her because, for a week, she had seen through the curious, delighted eyes of a child. She had gained what the Buddhist's call the "beginner's mind." Far from being stale, she was gripped with a child's curiosity which had made her more open, playful, and able to be surprised. She had reclaimed that childhood ability to see things as they really are, as if for the first time. As she stopped imposing her staleness on things, they began to reveal themselves to her in new and wondrous ways. She had become pure with the moment.

Perhaps the most difficult place to practice purity is with ourselves. Be honest, how many expectations and illusions do you impose on yourself? I am amazed when I read old journals and find them filled with all the things I will do to improve myself. When I listen to others talk, I know I am not the only one who is hoping to make myself into a picture-perfect version of me. Rather than planning ourselves, what if we practiced "unplanning" ourselves? Instead of striving to become someone lovable, what if we loved ourselves fiercely as we are? Instead of managing ourselves, what if we loosened the reins? The question remains for each of us to answer, "Can you be pure with yourself in each moment?" Or in the words of Anthony de Mello, "Can you leave yourself alone?"

> Being pure with ourselves means we are not afraid of our thoughts or our feelings, and we do not have to hide anything from ourselves.

Being pure with ourselves means we are not afraid of our thoughts or our feelings, and we do not have to hide anything from ourselves. Matthew Sanford, speaking from the experience of an accident that left him paralyzed from the waist down, says, "I am not afraid of my sadness. My sadness is an incredible gift that allows me to be with people who are suffering without trying to fix them." Matthew invites us to simply and fearlessly be with all the pieces of ourselves.

Being pure with all the pieces of ourselves increases our staying power with our own suffering, intimacy, joy, boredom, pain, and anxiety. We become safe with ourselves, and we become a safe place for others. We become a person who can comfortably and compassionately sit with another without the need to fix them.

Gathering the Scattered Pieces of Ourselves

Not only does purity ask us to subtract the illusions we impose on the moment, it also asks us to gather ourselves together so that our whole self shows up to the moment. What does this mean? Yogiraj Achala uses the phrase "be unalloyed." Alice Christensen speaks of being "unfragmented." Whatever term we use, purity asks that all of us be in one place at one time. And that means that our head and heart are unified, our thoughts, actions, and speech are congruent, and we are in the present moment.

One of my friends related an incident with her three-year-old son. It was a particularly busy day and she was attending to many different things. In the process of all her busyness, her son was trying to get her attention. Frustrated, he grabbed her face between his hands and said, "You're not recognizing me." As this little three-year-old reminded his mother, each moment, each person, each event, asks us to recognize it by truly being present to it as it is.

Like my friend in the story above, we often enter an

experience with the clutter of scattered thoughts and leave the experience with even more cluttered thoughts. It is like we are living on the leftovers of where we have been or the preparations of where we are going. Because we have not taken the time to "catch up" with ourselves, we are everywhere but the present moment. We are missing out on the fullness of life lived in the richness of what is immediately before us. Instead of entering the moment relaxed and spacious, we arrive frazzled and late because we tried to do one more thing before we left. And often we leave messy and cluttered, already rushing off mentally to our next thing instead of breathing in a sweet closure to the moment.

> Because we have not taken the time to "catch up" with ourselves, we are living on the leftovers of where we have been or the preparations of where we are going.

The practice of purity asks us to slow down and do one thing at a time. Purity embodies the slow steadiness and integrity necessary to give all of our attention to one thing at a time. As we practice slowing down and giving each thing our undivided attention, we will find ourselves more integrated and more pure with the moment. Hurrying, multi-tasking, and busyness, all symbols of success in our culture, are killers of purity.

I have had the experience of waking up to my morning prayers and meditation, only to find that in one line of a prayer, I have almost planned my entire upcoming day. I have also had the experience of looking lovingly into my granddaughter's eyes as she is about to speak and then realizing a moment later that she is finished speaking and I have not heard a word she said. In both of these instances, the moment happened and I was not there.

Purity requires all of our attention in the moment so that we can go on to the next thing with our full awareness and energy. Krishnamurti writes of the freedom this kind of engagement brings when he says, "I enter fully into each experience, and I come out fully from each of them too. I put the whole of me into all I do, and...out of all I do." Purity asks that we make full and honest contact with the moment so there is nothing lost and no regrets. There is no residue.

> Purity asks that we make full and honest contact with the moment so there is nothing lost and no regrets.

Several years ago I studied the Lord's Prayer in its original Aramaic language with Neil Douglas-Klotz. The line interpreted in English as, "...and forgive us our trespasses as we forgive others..." when spoken in Aramaic, has a spitting out quality, as if saying the line itself is a letting go. Douglas-Klotz interpreted this spitting out quality of the words as a literal act of forgetting what you know about the other person.* It is as if

---

*One literal translation of the Aramaic is "Loose the cords of mistakes binding us, as we release the strands we hold of others' guilt." Note also, that although the New Testament of the Bible is written in Greek, the language of the common people of that time was Aramaic. Jesus would have spoken the words of the Lord's Prayer and taught them to the people in Aramaic. Aramaic became a "dead" language in later centuries as the Muslims took power in the area and Arabic became the predominant language.

you meet each person with a clean slate, not remembering any secrets they may have shared with you. The hidden hope is that each time you see this person you can see them and relate to them in a pure manner. I often remember this line and notice that the secrets I know about others are mere clutter in my mind that keep me from the practice of purity. I continue to pray this petition of forgetting.

The practice of *Saucha*, or purity, of cleansing ourselves and cleansing our ability to be with each moment, takes on a visceral quality. As we begin to lose the heaviness of waste and clutter, we begin to feel lighter, more spacious and expansive. Our bodies become more alive, our minds become more clear, our hearts more compassionate. ❧

Questions for Exploration

Living with these questions, taking time for reflection, and journaling will give you new insights into your life and the practice of purity. For this month, frame your exploration in the following statement by Krishnamurti:

I enter fully into each experience,
and I come out fully from each of them too.
I put the whole of me into all I do,
and...out of all I do.

Week One: This week notice where your body is sluggish. Begin to purify yourself through diet and exercise (and the space around you if that is making you sluggish). Notice how the sluggishness becomes lighter as you purify. Notice the difference between the external process of cleansing and the internal process of purifying.

Week Two: This week, begin to purify your thoughts and speech. Use friends, ritual, forgiveness, journaling, etc. to release toxic, stale, negative thoughts. Replace these thoughts with love and gratitude.

Week Three: This week, be purely with yourself. In the words of Anthony de Mello, leave yourself alone. Journal the experience and what gets evoked for you.

Week Four: This week, set aside one undisturbed hour where you take the entire time to eat one orange. Give this orange, and the delight of eating it, your full attention for the whole hour. For the rest of the week, slow down and be purely with each moment as it presents itself. Journal your experience.

For this month ponder the words of Krishnamurti and live purely with each moment as it is. ॐ

SANTOSHA

Stay in the center
and notice each moment with
calm serenity.
~ C.L.

संतोष

संतोष

Santosha: Contentment

My husband and I own the three seasons of the TV series *Kung Fu* on DVD. We enjoy watching these episodes and pretending that, like Caine, we are masters of life; that no matter what happens, we can remain calm and know exactly what to do.

For those of you unfamiliar with the series, Caine, as a young orphan, entered a Chinese monastery and was trained in the martial arts and way of the Tao. He became a master in his own right and was initiated into a sect of the Buddhist priesthood. After an incident in which Caine was blamed for the death of the emperor's favorite nephew, Caine fled to America as a wanted man.

It is in America that we watch Caine wander from town to town in complete mastery of his own life. Bounty hunters are continuously after him, yet he does not walk in fear; instead he meets each moment with

Santosha invites us into contentment by taking refuge in a calm center, opening our hearts in gratitude for what we do have, and practicing the paradox of "not seeking."

curiosity and total presence. He has nothing but he does not walk in lack; instead he meets each moment satisfied, able to see beauty and abundance. Where most people would find loneliness and deprivation, Caine finds contentment. And in his contentment, he is able to skillfully invite others into a

119

deeper realization of their own ability to be strong of will and gentle of heart.

Contrast this image of contentment with a sweet story my friend told me about her childhood. She remembers as a little girl of six, standing on her front porch, gazing into the distance, and thinking to herself, "Somewhere, people are having so much more fun than I am." Perhaps you, like I, can see the innocence of longing coming from this small child. And yet, as we grow through the years of our life, it is this continued longing that keeps contentment out of our grasp.

In this country, advertisers magnify this longing in us, so that wanting what we don't have has become a contagious plague. Rather than experiencing contentment, we can find ourselves busy getting ready for the next thing, tossed about by our preferences for what we like and what we don't like, and riding the waves of annoying disturbances. The jewel of *Santosha* invites us into contentment by taking refuge in a calm center, opening our hearts in gratitude for what we do have, and practicing the paradox of "not seeking."

Always Getting Ready

There is a Chinese proverb which states, "People in the West are always getting ready to live." There is a remarkable truth to this proverb. When we are little we can't wait to get big, when we are big, we can't wait to get out of the house, then we can't wait to get through college and get a job, then we can't wait until our vacations, and finally, we can't wait until retirement. As the Chinese proverb states, we never really live, we just get ready.

संतोष

Along with getting ready for the next thing, we tend to look at other people's lives and see what is missing in our own. We look across the fence and see what we don't have, rather than look inside the fence and enjoy what we do have. When we look over the fence, we move ourselves into lack. A friend tells the story about how envious one of her sisters was of her during the time my friend led wilderness adventure trips. One day, the sister decided to go on one of these trips. On a particularly hard day she found herself sitting miserably on the beach. A cold wind was blowing through her and she was not feeling well from her monthly cycle. She looked at my friend and calmly said, "I'm not jealous of you anymore."

When we expect the world to meet our needs, we turn outside of ourselves to find sustenance and completion. We expect our partners to fulfill us, our jobs to meet our needs, and success to solve all of our problems. And when it doesn't, we continue to play the "if only" game, looking for that one more thing. Or we play the "planning" and "regretting" game. We let our contentment be managed by all these uncontrollable variables. As long as we think satisfaction comes from an external source, we can never be content. Looking outward for fulfillment will always disappoint us and keep contentment one step out of reach.

Pleasure & Avoidance

We spend vast amounts of our lives moving towards what we like, whether the object is food, clothes, colors, music, self image, conversation, hobbies, friends, activities, or beliefs. We see our preferences in all these areas as that which gives us pleasure and we seek the permanence of that pleasure in our lives like it was a matter of life and death. Likewise, we move away from what we don't like. Anything that puts our pleasure at risk we see as repulsive and to be guarded against.

We think we are free but in truth we spend huge amounts of our energy maneuvering ourselves and manipulating others so that our days will be filled with what we like and be void of what we don't like. I have noticed this maneuvering of life as a physical feeling of "gripping" in my body. When I find myself around something that gives me pleasure it is almost like something in me grips with the desire for that pleasure. The same gripping sensation happens when I think I might miss out on the pleasure. Likewise, when I find myself in a meeting feeling bored or restless, I feel tenseness inside my body as if I am trying to protect myself from the unpleasant experience.

> Looking outward for fulfillment will always disappoint us and keep contentment one step out of reach.

In truth, the yogis tell us, things are neutral. It is the personal labeling we put on these things that makes them appealing or repulsive to us. When I was a small child I was made to sit at the kitchen table and finish eating my plateful of squash. It took me several miserable hours to complete the task, after which I swore to hate squash for the rest of my life. For decades I carried on my hate campaign towards squash. It wasn't until very recently that I looked at a squash in the store with more curiosity than hatred. I boldly bought the squash, brought it home, cooked it, and ate it. Much to my surprise, I loved the taste! The point is that the squash was neutral. It was my long history of giving meaning to the squash that made it at differing times, both repulsive and pleasurable.

Seng Ts'an poignantly stated, "The way isn't difficult for those who are unattached to their preferences." If you want to begin to experiment with the truth of this statement, try spending days doing what you don't like and not doing what you do like and see how attached you are to your preferences. It is our need to satisfy our preferences that keeps us from contentment and makes our days difficult. Our seeking and avoiding (tensing and gripping) become expensive uses of our energy.

Oscar Wilde once said that there are two kinds of unhappiness in the world. One is *not getting* what you want; the other *is getting* what you want. Perhaps he knew that satisfying our likes and avoiding our dislikes just keeps us on a roller coaster of needing to continue to satisfy our likes and avoid our dislikes. True freedom and contentment begin to find their way to us when we can see things as they are, neutral, and not spend so much energy manipulating things according to our preferences. I am reminded of the wisdom of a 116 year old man, who, when asked the secret to his longevity, replied, "When it rains, I let it."

> Seeking and avoiding are expensive uses of our energy.

We are Responsible for our own Disturbances

Not only do we ride the waves of likes and dislikes, we also ride the waves of emotional disturbance. Think of how often you feel upset, hurt, left out, not appreciated, put upon, etc. It is easy to give the power of our emotional state to someone or something outside of ourselves. When we give away our emotional well being to what others are saying or not saying or to how the day is unfolding, we are at the mercy of things beyond our control; we have allowed our own contentment to be determined by what other people say or do; we have made ourselves helpless.

> When we give the power of our emotional state to someone or something outside of ourselves we have made ourselves helpless.

Carlos Castaneda writes, "Think about it – what weakens us is feeling offended by the deeds and misdeeds of our fellow men. Our self-importance requires that we spend most of our lives offended by someone." Whether we react to this perceived offense with a verbal explosion, silence and withdrawal, confiding in someone else, or saving the offense until six months later when no one else remembers, emotional disturbance is an inappropriate and wasteful use of energy. It is a stance of powerlessness that guarantees contentment will always be out of reach.

In my experience consulting with companies, private coaching with individuals, and in my own family life, it is clear to me that emotional disturbance takes a huge toll. It causes a loss in service to the client, unnecessarily sloppy work on the team, pain and misunderstanding in the family, and a toll on our own health and well-being. When we are hooked on our disturbances, we have tunnel vision and we regress to the level of intelligence of the emotional disturbance. When we are not

संतोष

hooked, we have access to a panoramic vision, we can see all the angles, we can see a clear win-win, creative direction.

As if outside events weren't enough to hook us into emotional disturbance, when things are quiet we can tend to play and replay stories in our minds that are sure to cause us to be upset. Whether we're remembering what someone did to us ten years ago or yesterday, the mind has an amazing ability to relive this disturbance over and over and over again, bringing us deeper and deeper into discontent.

There is a Japanese proverb that states, "The noise does not disturb you, you disturb the noise." I admit, as a lover of silence, I had to think about this for a long time. I have always viewed loud noises as disturbances of my "calm, peaceful" nature. What this proverb so brilliantly taught me is the reality that when I am upset by noise, I am the one who is disturbing the flow of life, not the noise! There is no escape; we can always trace our emotional disturbances back to ourselves. We keep ourselves out of contentment.

Much like emotional disturbances can easily hook us, the glitter and promises of the outside world also demand our attention. I especially noticed the stimulation of technology when I returned from a month Sabbatical in the woods. I wrote the following as I watched myself slowly move from a place of contentment to the captivating buzz of stimulation:

Ringing. That's what it was. On Sabbatical I never heard any ringing. No ringing of the doorbell announcing someone wanted to see me. No ringing of the telephone creating a duet with the programmed

ringing of my cell phone, often making
a trio of sounds as my computer would
chime in "mail truck," announcing at least
one new email has arrived, making a total
of at least three people who were trying
to contact me at the same time. Nor was
there the ringing of my alarm clock telling
me it was time to start the day or get up
from a nap.

Now that I am home, I am witness to the
cacophony of rings. Unlike the sounds of
nature where I could sit in pure delight
being drawn more and more inward in
contemplation, these rings are impatient
taskmasters jolting me from my present
state and demanding an immediate
response. Notice me now. Answer me
now. Attend to me now. Whatever I was
peacefully doing is now forgotten, my
attention now shifted to the "ring." And I
notice that my responses range anywhere
from total annoyance to the excitement
of an unknown Christmas package. Who
is on the phone? Who just emailed me?
Now what does someone else want from
me? The stimulation and demands are
constant and I begin to wonder, "Who is
running the show here?" If I'm not careful
I become a yoyo to my responses of the

various ringing sounds. A willing slave to drop whatever I am doing to respond to the ring. I am being trained to need stimulation and let a ring call me from my contentment. I am becoming one of Pavlov's dogs.

Gratitude

It is not easy in this culture to stay contented. So how do we get there and how do we stay there? I can spin out of contentment so quickly that I am caught off guard with the surprise of it all. I watched myself one particular morning and learned once again the need for gratitude as a tool to keep myself centered in contentment. I was visiting a friend and was suddenly overcome with the beauty and location of her home. The rumblings of discontent had begun. I hadn't traveled this pathway for quite some time, but now on it, I watched with amazement at how fast the terrain became steeper and steeper until I was at a dead run, tumbling down into the land of discontentment. Nothing was right with my life; nothing was right with me.

My morning began with meditation and a lovely visit to a friend's beautiful home. How did I end up here, bruised and disgruntled with the whole of my life? And how did I get here so quickly? One brief moment, a twinge of jealousy for someone else's home, and within an hour I had forgotten that I have a beautiful home, a rich life, a healthy vital body, a loving family, and a passion for life. I had imprisoned myself in lack.

I began to trace back my morning until I landed on a secret. Somehow gratitude had slipped out of my heart, leaving me vulnerable to the rumblings of discontent. I had reversed a formula in my head. Instead of being grateful for what I have and happy for my friend, I had slipped out of gratitude and into envy.

I discovered the secret of gratitude many years ago when life took me from my home town, Kansas City, to a town of one-hundred in eastern Montana. I did not have yoga skills at the time, nor had I honed a very grateful heart; the move felt harsh for a city girl. From a sunken place of despair, something creative and playful called out to me in the form of a challenge: "Let's play the thank you game," the voice said. I had no idea what the thank you game was, but I began to search hard for clues and cracks and pauses in which I could, with some kind of honesty, say thank you to life. What I discovered turned my world upside down. It wasn't long before my step was lighter and slowly almost everything began to bring a smile to my face and words of gratitude to my heart. I was alive again, and the small town was enchanting.

> Practicing gratitude protects us from our own pettiness and smallness and keeps us centered in the joy and abundance of our own life.

Practicing gratitude protects us from our own pettiness and smallness and keeps us centered in the joy and abundance of our own life. When stimulation pulls at us and disturbance beckons us, it is the gratitude uttered from our lips that keeps us strongly rooted in contentment.

Maintaining Center

The Buddhists speak of developing an abiding calm. A centeredness that is unshakeable. Like a tall tree so rooted in the earth that great winds cannot topple it. This for me is the image of contentment. It means not riding the waves of the ups and downs of life. It means that we not only agree to what is in the moment, but we actually welcome it. It means that in all the noise and demands of modernity, we stay in the abiding calm center. This is the mastery of life that contentment invites us into. The practice of gratitude and "nonseeking" can help us stay rooted in this jewel.

The Paradox of Not Seeking

There is a paradox to *Santosha*: The more we seek it or need it to look a certain way, the more it eludes us. I find that I am continually faced with my illusions of contentment. I have an image in my mind that I will always be centered and calm, that life will always seem perfect to me. It is, I think, this very image that keeps tripping me up and keeping me from the contentment I seek. Think about it, it is easy to be content when we feel great and things are going our way and we like ourselves. But what about when chaos and interruptions abound or we feel bored or depressed? What then?

Discontentment is the illusion that there can be something else in the moment. There isn't and there can't be. The moment is complete. That means if I am bored or sad, I will only be discontented if I am not content to be bored and sad. Building contentment with boredom, sadness, impatience, depression, disappointment, and loss, builds our ability to be that tall tree so rooted in the earth that great winds cannot topple it. Being content with our discontentment is itself a gateway to the calm depths within.

The paradox of not seeking contentment, allows us to appreciate what we have. Swami Rama stated it this way, "Contentment is falling in love with your life." In the beloved classic *The Wizard of Oz*, Dorothy embarked on a long journey to discover that she already had contentment where she was. In the words of Swami Rama, she had fallen in love with her life.

Santosha, or contentment, is performing duty and right action with pure joy. It is the true understanding that there is nothing more that can or does exist than this very moment. When we are purely in the moment, the moment is complete. When we do something in the moment to fulfill an expectation for another moment, for instance exercising to get our bodies to look a certain way rather than for the pure joy of movement, we will miss contentment. When action is complete in the moment, and the process is enjoyed for the pure joy of the process, action becomes being, and being becomes contentment.

> Discontentment is the illusion that there can be something else in the moment. There isn't and there can't be. The moment is complete.

I am inspired by reading mystics from all traditions. One of the things I notice is how they all love God – in whatever form they understand God. They never need approval from anyone because they are too busy having a love affair with God. The mystics are always content. Nothing can pull them out of contentment, because they see with eyes of love and wonder that keep them out of any kind of neediness.

Maezumi Roshi, a Zen master once said, "Why don't you die now and enjoy the rest of your life?" The mystics have "died" to their own needs, to their own wants and desires, to disturbances and stimulation, and now they can live fully in the tranquility of contentment. The mystics have learned that there is nothing missing; life is complete the way it comes to us in each moment. When we understand this, we sink into contentment. ✌

Questions for Exploration

Living with these questions, taking time for reflection, and journaling will give you new insights into your life and the practice of contentment. For this month, frame your exploration in the following statement by Swami Rama:

Contentment is falling in love with your life.

Week One: This week notice when you find yourself getting ready for the next thing or looking for contentment from something outside of yourself. Journal your observations.

Week Two: This week notice how much energy you expend moving towards what you enjoy and avoiding what you dislike. Notice any physical gripping sensations in your body. Journal what you notice.

Week Three: This week take responsibility for all your emotional disturbances. Trace every annoyance and upset back to yourself. Choose to stay in the disturbance or to return to the calm center of contentment (or to be content with your disturbance).

Week Four: This week practice gratitude and nonseeking. Be content with each moment as it is. Ponder these words from the mystic Meister Eckhart, "If the only prayer you say in your entire life is 'Thank you' that would suffice."

For this month ponder the words of Swami Rama and fall in love with your life as it is. ❧

TAPAS

*Can you show courage
and stay in the fire until
you find the blessing?
~ C.L.*

तपस्

Tapas: Self-Discipline

My husband talks about growing up on a large acreage outside of town. Periodically, to care for this land, his father would do a controlled burn. My husband watched as his father diligently prepared by checking the wind speed, wind direction, and the weather forecast for any unwanted or unforeseen surprises. And then my husband watched in disbelief as his dad lit a match to the field, and everything went up in flames. As a small child, none of this made sense to him, especially as he gazed at the stark after effects of the burn; everything looked charred and ruined. But within a few weeks, tiny green growth would sprout through the seemingly dead land, bringing new life and beauty, a kind of new beginning. My husband began to understand that the land had to be burned of its debris in order for it to produce its luscious bounty once again.

Tapas literally means "heat," and can be translated as catharsis, austerities, self-discipline, spiritual effort, change, tolerance, or transformation. *Tapas* has the sense of "cooking" ourselves in the fire of discipline to transform ourselves into something else. It is our determined effort to become someone of character and strength. Much like cooking an egg denatures the egg, changing it into a different structure, *Tapas* eventually changes our nature, turning us into

> *Tapas* is our determined effort to become someone of character and strength.

तपस्

a cauldron that can withstand any of life's challenges. *Tapas* is the day to day choice to burn non-supportive habits of the body and mind, choosing to forsake momentary pleasures for future rewards.

In India some spiritual renunciates practice extreme austerities. In the dead of winter they sit for three hours in the cold dressed only in a loincloth. They rig a container so that it will drip cold water on their heads and run down their almost naked bodies for the entire three hours. They do this practice for forty-five days in a row. In the heat of summer, they build five small fires around themselves and one in a container on their head. Then they sit for three hours in the blazing heat. They build these fires daily and sit for three hours for forty-five days. This is done to establish themselves in a firm, unmovable center that is not rocked or disturbed by any extremes the external world may bring. They practice staying still no matter what thoughts or fears are running through their own minds.

Our practice does not need to be this daunting; however, the example of these spiritual ascetics might inspire us to a little more depth in our discipline. And, much like a controlled burn, we need to pay attention to what is possible, what is safe, and what is timely for us in our current life context. When we have "tested the wind" we can light the match, willingly burning away our laziness and our selfish desires. Whether we practice *Tapas* by showing up at our mat for a regular posture practice or through constant acts of selfless service, we offer ourselves to the next higher version of us. We willingly stand the heat so that we might produce "luscious bounty" with our lives.

This guideline not only speaks to our personal effort,

but also to those cathartic times of almost hopeless desperation when we find ourselves in the pain of unexpected loss or debilitating sickness, or in the throes of a life that seems like it has been turned upside down. It is almost as if God has checked the winds and started the fire and we ourselves are the field that is being burned. And, like my husband who watched his father burn a field, none of it makes sense to us at the time.

> It is the times of hopeless desperation that shape and mold us into someone of depth.

And yet it is these times that shape and mold us into someone of depth. Our debris gets burned away and we are left more humbled and strengthened by the mystery of what is beyond our grasp of control or of understanding. It is these darkest times of pain, loss, and confusion that weave something profound in us.

Spiritual teacher Ram Das speaks eloquently to this jewel of *Tapas*. When he experienced a debilitating stroke, something he never expected to happen to him, he found a new opportunity for himself and for others as he began to wrestle with the possibilities and effects of aging. He chose to speak of his experience as "being stroked" by God, rather than as having had a stroke. And he termed the phrase "fierce grace" to speak of his experience of being burned by the fire of divine love.

There is a bumper sticker which states, "A crisis is a terrible thing to waste." We can chuckle all we want, but there is great truth to this statement. *Tapas* can take us to the place where all of our resources are used up, where there is nothing left but weakness, where all of our so-called "props" have been taken away. It is in this barren place, where we have exhausted all that we have and all that we are, that new strength is shaped and character is born if we choose to fearlessly open ourselves to the experience. It is perhaps the greatest gift life could offer us.

Charlene Westerman speaks truthfully to the danger and the possibility of catharsis when she states that during these times we have two choices: to break down or to break open. We can't prevent these times of catharsis in our lives or know their shape or outcome, but we can prepare ourselves for them through our daily practice, through building our ability to stay in unpleasantness, and through the small, daily choices we make.

Tapas as Daily Practice

When I lived near the shores of Lake Sacajawea, I had the grace of time to take long walks on miles of land that held the promise of seeing no one. One day I stumbled upon a large nesting site for blue herons along the banks of the lake. I became a constant visitor until the herons accepted me as part of what belonged. I watched as eggs were laid and tended; I watched as young chicks poked and maneuvered their way out of their shell homes, now become prison; I watched as these newborns were tended and fed. I watched as they grew to look more like herons than fuzzy masses. Finally the day came, when I was privy to their flying lessons.

It had never occurred to me that a bird wouldn't automatically know how to fly perfectly. What I watched was a comedy in errors. I watched the parents strategically fly off (but not too far) and leave the young ones seemingly unattended to figure flying out for themselves. I watched as the brave ones began to try their wings and hover ever so slightly above the nest. And then I watched them get braver and fly out of their nests and begin to play with the wind and landings. I watched as attempt after attempt was made to land back in the nest, only to be misjudged over and over again. Whoops! I don't think I have ever laughed so hard in my life, nor been so touched by the beauty of this mastering of flying.

Somewhere we forget that we had to learn how to walk, like these young birds had to learn to fly. We forget how many times we fell. We forget that things take practice. Ray Charles was asked later on in his career if he still practiced and prepared for concerts. He replied that he played scales everyday, because when the scales were in his fingers, he could play anything. The question becomes for us, what are we practicing for? When is the last time you even asked yourself this question?

> The question becomes for us, what are we practicing for? When is the last time you even asked yourself this question?

Our granddaughter Tiana, at the very young age of three, knew she wanted to be on stage as a singer and dancer. She forsook all kinds of childhood pleasures to practice for hours, mimicking her favorite singer's words, gestures, and dance steps. And then she would delight us by performing a perfect routine. Tiana understood that to become something in the future takes effort in the now.

In yoga, having a daily disciplined practice is referred to as *Sadhana** and is much like doing a small controlled burn on ourselves. It is the discipline of putting ourselves in places where the old debris that has collected in us can be removed. We engage in this process when we pay attention to the amount and kind of food we put in our body, when we move and exercise our bodies through walks, yoga, and other activities, when we expand our mental ability, or study scripture with like-minded people. This process begins to remove unwanted pounds, lazy habits, an unexercised heart and body, a stale mind, and an unheard spirit. As Pattabhi Jois reminds us, "Practice, and all is coming."

St. Francis of Assisi, in his well-known prayer, speaks eloquently to the possibilities of transformation for each human being.

Lord make me an instrument of thy peace.
Where there is hatred, let me sow love;
Where there is injury, pardon;
Where there is doubt, faith;
Where there is despair, hope;
Where there is darkness, light;
Where there is sadness, joy.

This is a profound plea to change us from haters to lovers and from disturbers of peace to makers of peace. This is the prayer of *Tapas*, and it invites us to be in life in a different way.

Sadhana means spiritual discipline. It implies a dual aspect that the discipline itself is the fulfillment. Like a drop of water eventually shapes a rock, the consistency of practice over a period of time brings the change and fulfillment. *Sadhana* is the consistency of our daily practice.

Tapas as Staying Power

One of my favorite stories in the Bible is the one that tells of Jacob wrestling with the Angel.* Jacob had had a bad day. Actually he had had a string of bad days since he cheated his brother out of the family birthright and had to flee for his life a great distance to find refuge with his Uncle Laban. After many years, Jacob returned home with wives, children, and livestock. As he got close to home, he saw his estranged brother with a band of warriors in the distance. This was the brother he had cheated. He figured he knew what was going to happen, and it wouldn't be pretty.

As things go when we're having a bad day, Jacob's day got worse. He had camped along a stream, by himself, when a stranger appeared and started fighting with him. You can almost hear Jacob say, "Good grief, what now?" Jacob had no choice but to fight back and the seemingly even match lasted until daybreak. Imagine Jacob's exhaustion – this on top of everything else.

At dawn the tide quickly turned, and Jacob realized the magnitude of who he was fighting with. It was someone of great power and strength who had merely been toying with Jacob all night. At this realization, instead of recoiling in fear and running for his life, Jacob did something quite amazing. He held on to this Being and begged for a blessing. Knowing full well the power of the Being, Jacob held on. And the Being, who had been wrestling Jacob all night, gave Jacob the blessing

---

*This story in the Bible is referred to as "Jacob wrestling with the Angel" but we never really know clearly who the Being is.

he sought. Jacob, in that moment renamed Israel* by the Being, was to be a great man, the leader of a great nation that would impact the world.

The Biblical text is vague in this passage. At the time, Jacob does not know who he is fighting with, nor do we. Is it a man, an angel, a supernatural being, God, Satan? Without knowing who or what has him in its grip, Jacob holds on until he knows he is blessed by the encounter.

So often we don't even know what has us in its grip; it seems dark and overpowering. In those times when we don't know how to get through the next minute of what seems unknown and overwhelming to us, can we, like Jacob, hold on? Can we hold on to what has us in its grip, gripping it back, and not letting go until we are somehow blessed by it? Can we grow our ability to stay in the fire and let ourselves be burned until we are blessed by the very thing that is causing us the pain and suffering?

> In those times when we don't know how to get through the next minute of what seems unknown and overwhelming to us can we hold on until we are somehow blessed by our struggle?

Jacob does not leave this scene with only a blessing. During the wrestling match, the Being had touched Jacob's hip, dislocating it. Jacob walked with a limp the rest of his life. Catharsis does not leave us untouched nor unscarred. We will be bearers of the wound, as well as the blessing.

St. John of the Cross writes meaningfully about *Tapas*

*The name Israel means "one who has striven with God and man and has prevailed."

in his treatise entitled *The Dark Night of the Soul.* St. John knew the harshness of catharsis when he found himself imprisoned in a monastery, treated with extreme deprivation and abuse by his fellow monks for his more liberal views. In his writings, he uses the example of a log being thrown into a fire to describe the process of being transformed by fire. He says that at first the log doesn't look anything like the fire and if the log has some impurities on the outside, the log will initially stink as it burns. But after a time, the log begins to look more and more like the fire, eventually becoming the fire itself.

Like Jacob, St. John of the Cross knew both the blessing and the resulting "limp," as the experience left him plagued with ill-health for the rest of his life. It also left him in constant communion with the Divine, for his dark night of catharsis had picked him up and taken him into the arms of God. *Tapas* is growing our ability to stay in the unknown and the unpleasantness, rather than run in fear. It is the willingness to be both burned and blessed.

> *Tapas* is the willingness to be both burned and blessed.

Tapas as Choice

A friend tells the story about leaving a partnership of eight years. At the same time she changed careers and moved to a new town; it was a daunting change for her. She writes, "I didn't start out with the clarity that I ended with. I started out not being able to breathe or eat. Struck with fear, anxiety and a feeling of being frozen, I needed to find something to help me move through the intensity of my life. My partner had a similar change. He too left the partnership, began a new career, and moved to a new town. He too, needed to find something to move through the intensity of this change. I found yoga and created a deep practice and did two-hundred sit ups a day. He chose drinking, smoking, and promiscuous behavior. At the end of that year of transition, our outcomes were very different. I had this silent strength that felt like it was emanating from my core; he was fragmented, exhausted and spiraling out of control."

> The promise of a crisis is that it will pick us up and deposit us on the other side of something. Will we trust the process or will we run and hide?

The story above is about the choices we make, in and out of crisis. If we, like my friend, can choose to strengthen our inner depth rather than medicate and run, we will find ourselves in a land of new possibility. Much like those turbulent teen years, where life has the awesome job of moving us from childhood to adulthood, the promise of a crisis is that it will pick us up and deposit us on the other side of something. Will we trust this process or will we hide from it?

Each moment is an opportunity to make a clear choice of right action. Quite often the choices that prepare us for the fire are options that vote against immediate satisfaction and pleasure. When we listen to our inner voice and surrender to staying present to the unknown, the unpleasant, and often to the grief and pain, we are preparing ourselves to benefit from and be blessed by *Tapas*.

Tapas

The discipline of *Tapas* will mold us into someone of great depth and profoundness if we let it. Can we stand the heat of being dismantled and changed forever by the fire? Can we prepare ourselves daily through our practice, our staying power, and our choices? Can we stay in the burning with integrity? Can we hold on for the blessing? ↷

तपस्

Questions for Exploration

Living with these questions, taking time for reflection, and journaling will give you new insights into your life and the practice of self-discipline. For this month, frame your exploration in the following statement by the mystic Rumi:

If you are a friend of God,
fire is your water.
You should wish to have
a hundred thousand sets of mothwings,
So you could burn them away,
one set a night.
The moth sees light and goes into fire.
You should see fire
and go toward light.
Fire is what of God is world-consuming.

Week One: Remember the cathartic times in your life and how you were shaped by them. Notice the times you may have "checked out" from the pain, and others where you were fearless in the fire and held on for the blessing.

Week Two: This week choose a practice of nourishing eating, meditating, contemplating, or something else that impacts the quality of your essence. Can you put yourself in the heat with enthusiasm?

Week Three: This week practice staying "one minute more" in whatever unpleasantness presents itself to you. Can you stand the heat of unpleasantness? Can you let the heat begin to burn away your judgments, opinions, and expectations?

Week Four: This week pay attention to your daily choices. Are you making choices that are indulgent, or making choices that build your strength and character? Listen to your inner voice and make choices that prepare you for the heat of life.

For this month ponder the words of Rumi and welcome the heat. ✍

SVADHYAYA

Know yourself so well
that you will grow into your
wholeness and greatness.
~ C.L.

स्वाध्याय

Svadhyaya: Self-Study

When my older brother and I were in grade school, we decided that our dad got cheated every Christmas by not receiving appropriate gifts for the love we felt for him. We decided to do something about that, and so, for a year, we saved all of our babysitting money and gift money until it was nearing Christmas. Then we had mom drop us off at a jewelry store where we proceeded to buy my dad the most beautiful diamond ring we could afford. We were delighted with ourselves.

When we got home, we decided such a gift needed to be wrapped in a special way. And so we set about gathering several boxes, seven to be exact, and, wrapping the diamond ring in its original box, proceeded to place it in the next size box, and then the next, until only one huge box remained. We wrapped the last box and placed it under the tree so our dad could spend the necessary time wondering what was in that huge box for him.

When Christmas arrived, my brother and I were beside ourselves with excitement. This was the day our dad would get his special gift that we had prepared for the whole year. He unwrapped the big box, only to find another box, and then another, and then another. Before too long, our dad had decided we were playing a grand practical joke on him and he moved into "good sport" mode, pretending to be exacerbated and delighted all at once. By the time he got to the last box, he was sure there was nothing waiting. But he was wrong. I don't think my brother or I will ever forget the look on his face when he opened that beautiful, sparkling diamond ring, purchased with the love of two adoring children.

The yogis teach that we, as human beings, are packaged much like this diamond ring. We are, at the core, divine consciousness. Around this pure consciousness, we are packed in "boxes" of our experience, our conditioning, and our belief systems. These boxes are things like how we identify ourselves, what we believe to be true, our preferences and dislikes, our fears and imagination. All of these boxes are informed

Svadhyaya, or self-study, is about knowing our true identity as Divine and understanding the boxes we are wrapped in. This process of knowing ourselves, and the boxes that adorn us, creates a pathway to freedom.

by country, culture, gender, town, ancestors and family history, groups we belong to, and our personal experience.

This packaging is portrayed in a story told in the East. It seems God had just created human beings. Realizing that He* had made a terrible mistake, God called a council of the elders to get some help. When the elders were gathered, God reported, "I have just created humans and now I don't know what I am going to do. They will always be talking to me and wanting things from me and I won't ever get any rest." Upon hearing God's dilemma, the elders made several suggestions telling God he could hide on Mount Everest, or the moon,

*In the East, God "being" is considered masculine, while God "acting" is considered feminine.

or deep in the earth. God responded hopelessly to all of these suggestions saying, "No, humans are resourceful; eventually they will find me there." Finally, one elder walked up to God and whispered something in his ear. Then God shouted in delight, "That's it! I'll hide inside of each human; they will never find me there!"

We suffer, the yogis tell us, because we forget who we are. We think we are the boxes we are wrapped in and forget that we are really the Divine "hiding" inside. *Svadhyaya*, or self-study, is about knowing our true identity as Divine and understanding the boxes we are wrapped in. We can find clues about our boxes by watching our projections, by the process of tracing our reactions back to a belief, and by courageously looking at life as it is. This process of knowing ourselves, and the boxes that adorn us, creates a pathway to freedom. The ability to shift our identification from our ego self (our "boxes"), to the witness, and finally to our true identity as Divinity itself, is the joy of this jewel of self-study.

Projections

Do this experiment now: without thinking, quickly write down the first five things that come to your mind that describe the world as you see it. Now look at what you have written. Every comment that you have used to describe the world will tell you more about yourself than about the world. You have just written clues into how you structure your beliefs, yourself, and your life. Every comment you make about the world, about another person, about an event, about life, is a projection of yourself and a clue to your interior landscape.

The world is your autobiography.

Let's return to the old *Kung Fu* re-runs. When Caine, fondly called Grasshopper by his master, is a small boy in the monastery, his master finds him watching fish in a small pond. The master asks Grasshopper, "How many fish are there?" Grasshopper replies, "Twelve, Master." "Good," replies the master, "and how many ponds are there?" Somewhat confused by such a seemingly obvious question, Grasshopper responds, "One, Master." "No," replies Master, "there are twelve ponds; twelve fish, twelve ponds." In the previous exercise, we could have asked a room full of five hundred people to do the experiment and all the answers describing the world would be different because each person would have described pieces of their unique self. Five hundred people, five hundred worlds.

The world and others simply reflect back to us what we are seeing, not what is there. It is as if wherever we look, there are only mirrors that show us pictures of ourselves. We cannot love or hate something about another person or the world unless it is already inside of us first. The world gives you what you see. You can experiment

> We cannot love or hate something about another person or the world unless it is already inside of us first.

with this truth by changing your story about what you see. You will notice, the world changes to fit the story you are telling.

The Buddhists say that the universe dies when you do because you have created your own little world of reality. As you begin to steadfastly pay attention to what you are saying to yourself about the moment, the other person, yourself, and life, you will get clues about the "boxes" you have wrapped yourself in that create your own little universe. All of these utterances are projections of the parts of yourself you love, don't love, can't see, or can't yet accept.

Tracing it Back

Usually we don't notice our beliefs or conditioning unless there is some kind of disharmony present. In these times, we have the opportunity to trace whatever we are saying about the moment back to a belief which we are either consciously or unconsciously holding. Tracing any disharmony back to ourselves will help us unpack a box we have ourselves wrapped in.

For instance, I come from a family of origin where we, as siblings, were not allowed to fight. Our family was about love, and loving meant we never fought. I carried that belief system, unconsciously, into my adult years. For me, when I saw anyone fighting, I judged it as wrong and interpreted it as meaning there was no love. By watching my judgment about fighting, I could eventually trace it back to this childhood belief, and begin to understand that some people show love for each other by fighting, and fighting wasn't necessarily "wrong." I was able to understand that people have different ways of showing love and affection. I was able to learn a new aspect about love, rather than staying firmly packed in the belief that love meant no fighting.

On a more recent occasion, I was at a retreat center where shoes were left at the door. On a break, I went to put my shoes on and they had disappeared. Shortly after, I saw another woman wearing them. I was not happy. I knew that I didn't really care if she wore my shoes, so I began to trace back what was disturbing me. I realized that I was mad because she hadn't politely asked to wear my shoes. In my childhood it was mandatory to say "please" and "thank you" before you took something; and if you forgot, you were punished. It was interesting to me that I wasn't bothered that she wore my shoes, but I was upset that she hadn't done what was "right" according to my belief system. In this incident, I was able to see the power of my unexamined beliefs.

> I was upset that she hadn't done what was "right" according to my belief system.

Our conditioning and formation of beliefs begins very early in childhood. Recently I watched as a group of young children emerged out of school for recess. I heard one child yell, "Freedom at last!" I chuckled but couldn't help wondering how this child's belief would further develop and influence the rest of his life. We learn early to accept our family's way of doing things and to pattern ourselves after cultural norms. These early conditionings continue to form and move deep inside us creating pieces of our identity. Add to that our reactions to our own life experiences and we become neatly wrapped in layers of packaging.

When faced with any disharmony, our tendency is to blame what is outside of us and then justify what we are thinking or feeling. If we are courageous enough to trace the disharmony back to ourselves, we can begin to unpack our boxes and open up vast amounts of freedom that brings us closer to our true essence. "Tracing it back" begins to unpack belief systems of "shoulds," "musts," and "wrong and right."

Anthony de Mello calls these belief systems "models of reality." He states, "We are happy when people/things conform and unhappy when they don't. People and events don't disappoint us, our models of reality do. It is my model of reality that determines my happiness or disappointments." It is as if we wrap ourselves in the boxes of our belief systems and conditioning and then, when something doesn't conform to our system, we fight with all our energy to justify our system, rather than to "unpack" the box. De Mello's message is that when we fight to keep our belief system, it is as pointless as if my Dad had wanted to keep his Christmas present wrapped and never open it to see the gift waiting inside.

Like a gift waiting to be opened, every event that life presents to us is a precious opportunity to learn the truth about the boxes we have ourselves packaged in. And it is especially the people "we can't stand" and the interruptions that "drive us crazy" that hold the greatest potential for us. Anthony de Mello put it like this, "Every time I am disturbed, there is something wrong with me. I am not prepared for what has come; I am out of tune with things; I am resisting something. If I can find out what that something is, it will open the way to spiritual advances."

We can't be Afraid to Look

We need our eyes and hearts wide open to look at every ripple of disharmony that we experience. Another school massacre has just occurred as I write this, and it is the bloodiest yet. The world is full of pain and suffering and deeds of horror. As I look back on my life, it is the pictures of starving children in Africa, the carnage of soldiers in the Vietnam War, the loss of hope on a Nicaraguan mother's face, which have shaped my heart and moved me to compassionate action. If we hide the pictures and the reality from ourselves, how can our hearts grow? If we close our eyes, our very lives rest on a false foundation. We can't be afraid to look.

We need our eyes and hearts wide open to look at every ripple of disharmony that we experience.

In my travel of third world countries, I have noticed how little is hidden. The old, the sick, the dying, the hungry, are not shut away like they are in this country. The guideline of *Svadhyaya* invites us to do the same with ourselves; not to shut the unpleasant parts of ourselves away, but to carry them with kindness and compassion, knowing that God lives there too.

I remember when Gandhi was interviewed by a reporter who asked him if he ever got incensed and outraged at his oppressors. Gandhi solemnly replied that no, he didn't, because he knew what existed in the interior landscape of his own being. He was not afraid to look at the fullness of emotions inside himself, and because of that fearless act of witnessing his inner being he was able to maintain courage rooted in kindness and compassion. Gandhi knew that denial cuts us off from the full reality of ourselves.

There is a Cherokee story in which the grandfather is explaining to his grandson that two animals live inside his heart, a wolf and a lamb. When the grandson asks what he is to do, the grandfather replies, "Feed the lamb." This story beautifully illustrates the reality of what sits inside us. We need to respect the wolf in us; if we don't, we may become self-righteous and vulnerable to being eaten by the wolf. Whatever we pretend isn't there will unconsciously use us. But we can choose to feed the lamb and grow ourselves into someone more compassionate and kind to both ourselves and to others. We must be willing to look at the selfishness and greed and anger that lies in us, but feed the greatness.

The Role of the Ego

The ego is a function of the mind that organizes itself into "I." The ego is not a bad thing; without the ego, we wouldn't exist. The ego takes an event that the senses bring into awareness and makes it personal. For instance, the senses may bring in the information that a dog is barking. The ego makes it personal by saying, "I hear a dog barking." Then, this message further gets entangled with the value judgment we place on the event. We will have an opinion about the dog barking based on our experience. I might be annoyed at the noise or tremble in fear because of a past experience where I was attacked. Or I might rush to pet the dog, remembering a childhood pet that I adored. We can see from this example how the ego takes ownership of a neutral experience by making it "mine" and then colors it from the box of past experience.

The above process is how the mind is designed to function so that we can have the experience of separateness; it is the ego that allows the experience of a walk in the park, the taste of fine chocolate, or a telephone conversation with a friend. Where things get messy is when the ego forgets that its function is to organize the self and begins to believe itself to be the boss. When this happens, we get stuck in the "I" of being separate, and we make our belief system the model of reality. Our belief system is not wrong or right, but it is constraining; when we identify with these constraints, we run on old habits and we consent to being less than we are.

As we unpack the boxes of our belief system, strong and often painful emotions can be released in the process. These feelings are often related to memories that we have unconsciously used to structure our reality. Similar to returning from a trip, where we have to take each item out of our suitcase and look at it as we unpack, we have to look at each box and the hidden emotions of experience that led to each layer of protective wrapping around ourselves. My experience is that the release can be quite unpleasant and I sometimes feel like I am swimming in muck. But I know that what might appear discouraging in the moment is often a cleansing release in disguise, an unpacking so to speak.

> As we unpack these boxes of our belief systems, strong and often painful emotions can be released in the process.

The path of growth is not a straight line; it does not look anything like what we think it should look like. In fact, often our belief system of what growth looks like, is the very thing that stops our growth. What we think we know stops our inquiry. The Buddhists remind us to have a beginner's mind; to know that we don't know. It is this stance of humility that opens the door to learning and revelation.

The ability to bring the witness into play in our lives is the ability to step outside of ego limitation and find out there is something more. It is to find that you are a soul, and then to polish the ego so that the ego becomes a function of the soul rather than a function of itself. Swami Veda writes, "It is by surrendering the limitations of its own banks that a river becomes the mighty ocean; do not be afraid to throw away the trinkets of your ego to gain the diamond of grace." This process begins with growing our ability to witness.

The Power of the Witness

I remember when our grandson Tyson was a toddler. Whenever he was asked by his parents to do something he didn't want to do, he would immediately switch to the third person, shifting his identity away from himself. He was always an "I" unless asked to do something against his wishes, in which case he became a "he." If his dad told him it was time to go to bed, Tyson would reply, "He don't want to." And then Tyson would continue to play, totally confident that as long as he didn't personally identify with it, he didn't have to comply with his dad's directive.

Watching Tyson switch back and forth between "I" and "he" was amazing to me as well as quite humorous. And yet, Tyson understood at this very young age, the power of distancing himself from himself. This power of the witness, to distance ourselves from ourselves, is how we begin to see how we have made up our realities. And paradoxically, it is how our belief system begins to lose its power over us.

Culturally, we are shaped to constantly engage in fixing

and analyzing ourselves (and others). As I watch myself and listen to others talk, I find this to be fundamentally true. I am always hearing things like: "If I just fix this, then I'll be OK" or "I know this isn't a very good thing about me, but I'm working on it." It seems we all have an obsession to fix ourselves and our attention is wrapped up in our shortcomings.

In western culture, we tend to analyze, fix, and control just about everything. If we don't like something about ourselves or our lives, we keep trying to figure out what is wrong and then fix it, all the while maintaining control to keep things as smooth as possible (translation: keep things the way we like them). Eastern thought has a different idea about this: East parts ways with the West at the point of needing to understand and fix. It is here that Eastern thought introduces the idea of "the witness."

The witness is our ability to watch ourselves act and respond. It is our ability to watch our thoughts and our emotional disturbances. This ability is what gives us clues into our matrix of belief systems. It is how we know ourselves and the stories that run us. The witness is our ability to watch the ego rather than identify with it. The profoundness of this watching is that we begin to know ourselves as something different than who we thought we were. It is this ability to watch that begins to bring healing to our lives.

> The witness is our ability to watch ourselves act and respond. It is this ability to watch that begins to bring healing to our lives.

Yoga's Upanishads talk about two birds in a tree. One is busy flitting around from tree to tree; the other sits on the limb watching. As long as we identify ourselves with the bird flitting around, we will be stuck in our belief system. The more we identify with the bird who simply watches, the more we will begin to understand our belief system. And it is the understanding of how we have created our reality that marks progress in our growth. Seeing our conditioning is the victory. Knowing that we aren't who we thought we were begins to open up the possibility of knowing our true Self.

> Knowing that we aren't who we thought we were begins to open up the possibility of knowing our true Self.

Yogiraj Achala tells the story about taking his young son to the Mississippi River. The son, looking into the river, asked his dad if the river was polluted. Yogiraj responded that no, the river is only carrying the pollution, the river itself is pure. Our minds are like the river carrying things in it. If we identify with what the mind is carrying–thoughts, stories, beliefs–then we will think we *are* those things. However, if we identify with the Divine within us (the pure river) and merely watch the thoughts float by, we will know we are simply carrying the thoughts, stories and beliefs; they *are not* who we are.

In another writing of Yoga's Upanishads, humans are referred to as "God in a pot." Understanding this simple statement is the goal of self-study. As long as we identify with the "pot" (our bodies and our minds), we suffer in our limitations. When we shift our identity from the "pot" to the

Godself within, we rest in our true Self. This Godself within is called the Atman in Yoga, Buddha nature in Buddhism, and Christ consciousness in Christianity.

Meditation is an important aspect of self-study; it is a place where we grow the witness, recognize our belief systems, and begin to shift our identity from the "pot" to the Godself within. Reading sacred scripture and inspirational biographies are other practices that bring us closer to our true identity. Engaging curiosity and a beginner's mind, knowing that we don't know, helps us step outside our neatly wrapped boxes. As we shift our attention to the Godself within, the boxes of belief systems begin to fall away, and we become free. ৎৎ

Questions for Exploration

Living with these questions, taking time for reflection, and journaling will give you new insights into your life and the practice of self-study. For this month, frame your exploration in the following statement by Huston Smith:

> We all carry it within us;
> supreme strength,
> the fullness of wisdom,
> unquenchable joy.
> It is never thwarted
> and cannot be destroyed.
> But it is hidden deep,
> which is what makes life
> a problem.

Week One: Ninety-nine percent of what bothers you is about you. Ninety-nine percent of what bothers others has nothing to do with you. This week notice how you turn the above statement around, blaming others for your own problems and taking responsibility for others' problems. Practice taking responsibility for yourself and letting others be responsible for themselves.

Week Two: This week notice what you project onto others. These projections are things you are unwilling or unable to acknowledge in yourself. Remember, you can't notice something in another person if it is not already in you (both your pettiness and your magnificence). Grow into full responsibility for yourself.

Week Three: This week, discover some of the boxes you have yourself wrapped in. Do this by tracing all ripples of disharmony back to yourself. Notice what personal belief system caused the disharmony. Is your belief true? Are you experiencing reality or a box? Support your efforts with these words from Anais Nin, "We don't see things as *they* are, we see things as *we* are."

Week Four: This week grow the power of your witness by watching all your actions and thoughts as if you were watching a movie. Begin to experience yourself as "supreme strength, the fullness of wisdom, unquenchable joy."

For this month ponder the words of Huston Smith and "unwrap" yourself. ℰ✤

Ishvara Pranidhana

Jump into your life
with your whole heart, trusting that
you will fly to God!
~ C.L.

ईश्वर प्रणिधान

Ishvara Pranidhana: Surrender

In the movie *Dirty Rotten Scoundrels,* two con men find themselves in the same lucrative area. Realizing that there is room for only one of them, they make a wager, agreeing to pick an innocent woman and con her out of $50,000. The first one of them to succeed in obtaining the $50,000 will maintain sole rights to "work" the area; the other will leave, never to return. The wager unleashes a comical set of events, in which each con man tries to out do the other. But the real surprise comes at the end, when it is the woman who swindles $50,000 from both of them! What is interesting to me are the reactions of these two men when they realize that all the time they thought they were doing the conning, in reality, they were being conned. In a fit of anger, one of the men reacts with what looks like a two-year-old tantrum. The other man, however, is very quiet and slowly begins to get a broad smile across his face. Then he begins to laugh in delight at the mastery of this woman who has outsmarted him and walked off with his $50,000.

There is a lesson for us here, I think. How often do we, like the men above, try to con life as if there is a prize waiting for us if we succeed? And when life doesn't do what we want, we throw a tantrum. (Just think about how many times you tell yourself you had a "bad day" because it didn't go the way you had planned.) We can be so busy feeling cheated or victimized when life doesn't go the way we want it to that we often miss a new opportunity life is offering us in the moment.

Ishvara Pranidhana, the jewel of surrender, presupposes that there is a divine force at work in our lives. Whether we call it God, grace, providence, or life, this force is greater than we are and cares deeply about us. Surrender invites us to be active participants in our life, totally present and fluid with each moment, while appreciating the magnitude and mystery of what we are participating in. Ultimately this guideline invites us to surrender our egos, open our hearts and accept the higher purpose of our being.

> *Ishvara Pranidhana,* the jewel of surrender, presupposes that there is a divine force at work in our lives. Ultimately this guideline invites us to surrender our egos, open our hearts and accept the higher purpose of our being.

We have had tastes of this jewel of surrender; we know it as being "in the flow" or "in the zone." In the movie *Bagger Vance*, it is portrayed as your "one perfect swing." Perhaps you were watching a sunset, hiking in the mountains, holding a baby, or caught up in something you love to do when suddenly time disappeared and you disappeared with it. Your actions, your thoughts, and the activity you were engaged in, lined up and became one entity of harmony and perfection. This is the rhythm of surrender. The yogis tell us that we can live this way all the time, unless we are getting in our own way.

Life wants to surprise, delight and grow us in ways far beyond our imagination. Jean-Pierre de Caussade understood the opportunity that hides in each event. In *The Sacrament of the Present Moment,* he writes about taking advantage of the "immense, certain, and always available good fortune" of every moment. He further states that there is a purpose hidden in each event, and if we trust this hidden purpose, life will always surpass our own expectations. De Caussade's writing overflows with the joy of trusting and finding God hidden within each activity, challenge, and interruption life presented to him.

How do we begin to find this rhythm of surrender or the immense joy and trust that overflows in the writings of de Caussade? When we release our rigidity and our need to control, when we joyfully engage life as it comes to us, and when we place our egos in devotion to that which is greater, we can begin to taste the bounty of this jewel.

Releasing

The yoga posture called *shavasana*, or corpse pose, is a posture for practicing surrender. Putting ourselves on our backs, with our arms and legs stretched out at a forty-five degree angle from the body, signifies the death of the activity we have just participated in. It is also a practice for the ultimate surrender of our own death. In *shavasana*, there is nothing for us to do. We are asked to just lie there, releasing any tension in our bodies, letting go of effort, and trusting that the breath will breathe us and the body will renew itself. (If this sounds easy, it's not.) This practice of *shavasana* is one of the most important practices we can do, for it is here that we begin to learn the meaning of letting go of all the ways we physically and mentally fight with life.

As we learn to stop fighting life, we can begin to act skillfully. Control makes us rigid and tight and narrows our perspective. Getting rid of our armor opens a world of possibility and makes us lighter and more comfortable for the journey. We can monitor our moment to moment surrender to life by watching the inner sensations of contraction and expansion. Contraction is a feeling of constriction, a pulling in. Expansion is an opening, a creating of space and wonder. When we find ourselves in contraction, we are fighting life or fearful of life. When we find ourselves in expansion, we are in the flow of surrender.

Doug Keller uses the imagery of ice chunks to help us grasp this concept of expansion and release. He likens life to a flowing stream and we are ice chunks in that stream. We are the same quality as the stream; however, we are frozen in our tensions and fears. Our practice is to melt ourselves into the flow of the stream, becoming one with the flow of life. As we relax and release our rigid thoughts and muscles, we can begin to flow with life.

When my granddaughter Ashly was a toddler I used to tell her to "be careful." In her delightful innocence, she mixed up the ending, and would always cheerfully reply, "Be care*free.*" I thought this was cute, and began to playfully mimic her. But I noticed something important as I shifted my language. I noticed that being careful created tightness in me; fear and rigidity accompanied these words. I also noticed that speaking the words "be carefree" brought an immediate feeling of expansion and opened me to the adventure of my life. I was ready to trust the moment.

> As we learn to stop fighting life, we can begin to act skillfully.

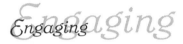 Engaging

Those of you who do white water rafting know the power of the rapids. To fight them is to lose. Instead, you must use the rapids to your advantage to navigate through them safely. Learning to surrender is as skillful as being able to maneuver a raft through white water rapids, knowing that the power is in the current and the rocks and your own skill to keep from capsizing or crashing. Like white water rafting, surrender is learning to skillfully ride with what the moment gives us, all the while enjoying the process, whether we glide through safely or tip over and get wet.

And yet, we can easily find ourselves waging war on the moment by demanding that it give us what we want, served just the way we like it. It would be like trying to make the current do what we want it to. That attitude is disastrous on a raft, and it is disastrous in life. When we need life to be a certain way, we get restricted and tight, rather than open to the current of life. But each time we ride the rapids, we become a more skillful paddler.

When discussing the first guideline of nonviolence, I talked about little three year old Brooks who began to hold his stools, creating internal discomfort for himself and disturbance for the whole household. There is more to the story. Brooks had started attending a new day care and was uncomfortable with one of the child care workers, whom Brooks referred to as "crabby." Brooks did not know how to handle the situation so he did the only thing he knew how to do at the time, hold his stools. But his mother Ann, aware of Brooks' fears with the situation, was able to invite him to walk through these fears. She took Brooks' courageous little hand, walked him up to an encounter with the child care worker, and stood by him while he came face to face with the person he feared. After this brave confrontation, Brooks was free, the childcare worker and Brooks became good buddies, and the house was back to normal.

The story above is an example of the power we have to meet life with courage and action. There was no denial of the severity of what was happening, nor was there a passive helplessness to the situation. Ann supported her son Brooks to meet life as it was, scary and overwhelming. And in the process, Brooks became more skillful in his relationship with life.

The story of Dietrich Bonhoeffer is another example of engaging the moment with integrity. Bonhoeffer was a Lutheran minister during the time that Hitler came into power. While others chose to ignore what was happening, Bonhoeffer stayed present to the reality of the moment. As he witnessed the atrocities of racism and fascism, he felt called to surrender to his need to act upon the suffering he was seeing. In a gut-wrenching decision, he became part of a small group of people who planned an assassination attempt on Hitler's life. The attempt failed, and Bonhoeffer was imprisoned. Just hours before Germany was liberated, Bonhoeffer was hung on the gallows. His writing during his days in prison while waiting for his own execution produced brilliant insights into the struggle, integrity and courage that life can demand of us. Surrender is not passive.

Engagement with the moment cost Dietrich Bonhoeffer his life. With Brooks, it demanded his courage. With others, such as William Wilberforce, whose passion and tireless efforts ended the British slave trade, surrender demanded his perseverance. History is full of great people who surrendered to the hardships and challenges of their time and engaged those hardships with creativity and skill. These inspirational people understood that surrender meant giving themselves to a higher purpose because that was what life asked of them. These people did not start out "great." Like you and I, they were ordinary people. But with each challenge life presented them, rather than shrink away, they grew themselves up to meet the moment skillfully.

Accepting

This is not to say that we should go looking for greatness, but rather to pay attention to the needs of the moment. If we are aware of what is right in front of us, we will get clues into our own development and direction. When life needs us, it will come to us, but we will recognize it only if we are paying attention and if we are courageous enough to respond. It is as if we are partnered to life in a dance step. We do not lead, nor do we limply drag along like dead weight. As a dance partner to life, we are asked to be vulnerable and undefended, and yet so present we can follow the next move, wherever the leading step takes us, adding our own style as we go.

Life knows what to do better than we do. Our task is simply to let go and receive each moment with an open heart, and then dance skillfully with it. If we have been practicing the other nine guidelines, we are learning to find our compassion and courage, our boldness and contentment, and the knowledge of how we get in our own way. As we grow in all the skills that the *Yamas* and *Niyamas* ask of us, we will be able to greet each moment worthy of what it asks of us.

Swami Rama used to say, "Do what is yours to do; don't do what is not yours to do." How simple these words may sound to our ears, and yet they are profound to our understanding of surrender. As we are able to let go of what we can't change, we are able to grow more and more into our unique gift and contribution to life itself. There is something that is ours to do, and whether it is large or small, it is our contribution to the whole of humanity. As we discern where our path lies and then surrender to that awareness, we will begin to taste freedom and joy in a way we never dreamed possible.

> Surrender asks us to be strong enough to engage each moment with integrity while being soft enough to flow with the current of life.

There is an image from the East that portrays the invitation of the tenet of surrender. The image is of a serpent so strong and balanced that it holds the entire earth on its head. Yet, it is soft enough for royalty and babies to be pampered as they lie comfortably on the coiled body. This is an image of strength and softness at *the same time*. Surrender asks this of us. To be strong enough to engage each moment with integrity and at the same time to be soft enough to flow with the current of life.

Devotion

A friend shared a vivid dream that had impacted her greatly.

In this life-like dream, a woman appeared to her and, popping out her chest, boisterously proclaimed, "The way to have a good day is to open up the door and LET GOD IN!" What a profound way to start each day in the remembrance and rhythm of surrender.

Surrender is ultimately a stance of devotion that takes place in the heart and permeates all of our attitudes and actions. In its deepest sense, *Ishvara Pranidhana* is the surrender of the ego to a higher purpose. Or, as Richard Rohr says, "It is the prayer of Thy kingdom come; my kingdom go." As the ego surrenders, the heart expands. As the ego stops working so hard to get its own way, life begins to take on an ease and rhythm. As the ego stops fighting to be number one, life begins to nourish and feed us in amazing ways.

> *Ishvara Pranidhana* is the surrender of the ego to a higher purpose. As the ego stops fighting to be number one, life begins to nourish and feed us in amazing ways.

As we grow ourselves into the fullness of what this jewel has to teach us, we begin to understand the magnanimity of what guides, protects, nourishes, and cares for us. We begin to understand that there is something much greater which is "doing" us, and we begin to give all of our actions, as well as the fruits of our actions, into the arms of the Divine. Surrender is knowing ourselves to be a part of this Divine Oneness and then giving ourselves over to this greater whole. We find in the process that we do not lose ourselves, but instead become part of the greatness itself. ☙

Questions for Exploration

Living with these questions, taking time for reflection and journaling will give you new insights into your life and the practice of surrender. For this month, frame your exploration in the following statement by Swami Chetanananda:

Ultimately there is nothing I can tell you
about surrender except
Having nothing and wanting nothing;
Not keeping score,
Not trying to be richer,
Not being afraid of losing;
Not being particularly interested
in our own personalities;
Choosing to be happy,
no matter what happens to us.
These are some of the clues.
The rest we learn with practice and grace.

Week One: This week watch your attitude and responses to the moment. Are you fearful, trusting, fighting, judging, or annoyed? Notice if there is a pattern to your attitude.

Week Two: This week notice any tension that arises in your body when you need the moment to be "your way." Consciously choose to relax your body and shift your attitude to curiosity. Notice what happens.

Week Three: This week practice welcoming each moment and growing yourself into the opportunity of what is being offered and asked of you. When you find yourself shrinking away, trust that life is giving you a chance to step into a fuller, more skillful you. Support yourself with these words from Pablo Picasso, "I am always doing that which I cannot do, in order that I may learn how to do it." Become a skillful, worthy student of each moment that life presents to you.

Week Four: This week wake up every morning and "let God in." Believe in something that is greater than you are and let your actions, your mind, and your heart line up with that greatness.

For this month ponder the words of Swami Chetanananda and learn about surrender through "practice and grace." ෴

Reviewing the Niyamas

Several years ago I made a major change in my life. Events came together in such a way that I asked myself the question, "Just how good can I feel?" I began to wonder if every year I could feel better and have more vitality and clarity. At the time, this question felt radical to me as I looked around at the American expectations of aging. But I decided it was worth the experiment and that I would make choices in diet, activity, and thinking that would support this exploration.

The *Niyamas*, or observances, are an invitation into a radical exploration of possibility. Just how good can you feel? Just how joyful can your life be? We will never know unless we consciously make choices to support this exploration. The five *Niyamas* outline the shape of these choices.

There is not a "right and wrong" to this exploration, nor is there a "better and worse." Like the *Yamas*, the *Niyamas* point us in the direction of something better than we are now aware of. It is as if we have five seeds to plant and care for in our inner being. They are the seeds of Purity, Contentment, Self-discipline, Self-study, and Surrender. We tend these seeds by:

- Cleansing our bodies, our speech, our thoughts
- Falling in love with our own life
- Consciously choosing discipline and growth
- Knowing the Self
- Paying attention to what life is asking of us

As these seeds begin to bear fruit, we will become unshakable as we experience an inner essence of deep harmony and strength and access to joy that bursts forth with every breath. The *Niyamas* are both the invitation and the guideline for this exploration. ℘

Purity	Invites us to cleanse our bodies, our speech, our thoughts.
Contentment	Invites us to fall in love with our own life.
Self-discipline	Invites us to consciously choose discipline and growth.
Self-study	Invites us to know the Self.
Surrender	Invites us to pay attention to what life is asking of us.

Moving On

As a child, I loved pretending I was a horse. Not just any horse, but a beautiful, black, fast horse, freely galloping over open countryside and taking giant leaps over anything in my way.

Although my relationship with horses has remained in my imagination, I still love them. They are beautiful animals and I brim with the thrill of watching them race with strength and grace on an open field or take those beautiful leaps in equestrian competition. The theologian Peter Marty, in speaking about equestrian competition, had some interesting observations. He stated, "Those of us whose only contact with the world of equestrian competition is via the television set find the elegance and ease of those leaping beasts to be almost surreal. We marvel at the calmness of the riders. We admire the cool focus as they vault their way over the hurdles [and wonder if those riders have] some extra instinct that the rest of us lack."

Marty further went on to talk about equestrian training. He noted that one of the most common obstacles all riders face is their own perception. Much time in training is devoted to the skill of the rider's own perception. It is known in the equestrian world, that unless a rider can approach these upcoming barriers with a kind of "anticipatory confidence," they will never be able to make these great leaps with their horses. Peter noted that one trainer put it this way: You have to "take your heart and throw it over the fence. Then jump after it."

We began this book with the premise that we are all engaged in the task of learning to become more fully human. As we look inside ourselves and outside at the world, we can see the immensity of this task. These are interesting times we find ourselves in. The polarities of our humanity seem like they are lit up in neon signs that we can't miss. We are witness to acts of brutality and greed that baffle our sensitivities and bring horror and disbelief to our hearts. We are also witness to acts of extreme compassion and kindness that inspire us with the potential that burns to be known in each one of us.

As I look at the world, it feels to me like we are trying to make a big choice about who we are as humans. And each one of us is part of this choice. The question then becomes, are we ready? Are we ready to grow ourselves into the best that Spirit can be, as it knows itself contained in a human body? Are we able to imagine days, and lives, and systems, and community the way a fully realized human would live them? Are we able to put our lives and our skill into bringing about this kind of world within us and around us? Are we able to "take our hearts and throw them over the fence and then jump after them?"

I think being a human being must be one of the hardest and most exciting adventures we could ever be engaged in. In this experience, we get to relish the taste of fresh strawberries and ice cream, melt into a lover's embrace, marvel at a child's innocent eyes, and delight in hikes in the woods and along beaches. We also get to weep deep wells of sorrow and grief and feel gusty torrents of rage and anger. Out of this vast continuum of emotions ranging from fear to compassion, we are capable of actions that impact the lives of others in rippling effects that would probably surprise us. We are bringers of suffering and light to this world in profound ways. This is an amazing reality that we need to affirm and then use skillfully.

Lest we think the task too great for us, Ann Maxwell reminds us that it is the daily choices that we must pay attention to. She writes, "It is relatively easy to be kind, compassionate, open, and expansive sitting on the safety of my yoga mat. I can be deeply in love here. I can offer my practice as a prayer. But the question remains, will I choose love once I step off this mat? The true test of love comes in the moment to moment ordinariness of life. Will I remain open as I walk back to my car in the dark? Will I find compassion in the face of judgment, both yours and mine? Righteousness, both yours and mine? Will I keep the love connection with my breath when I am running behind? Will I choose faith when my loved ones are in need? Will I be kind with house chores? Interruptions? These are the moments that our choices of fear or of love are most challenging and crucial."

To meet these daily tasks of living and larger visions for humanity, perhaps we, like equestrian riders preparing to take those big leaps, can be served by studying our own perception. Perhaps we could all use a boost of anticipatory confidence. Perhaps we need to trust those big and little leaps ahead of time and "throw our hearts over the fence....then jump after them."

The *Yamas & Niyamas* are the foundation for studying our own perception and for boosting our anticipatory confidence as we deal with the challenges and joys of our collective and singular humanity. May you know the power of these ten jewels to guide and shape the integrity of your life as you embark on this grand human experiment. ✆

Appendix 1

A Western vs. an Eastern Lens

Cultures have certain assumptions and unspoken "laws" about how to view life. These are not necessarily right or wrong, however, they do color that culture's experience of reality.

As Eastern concepts of yoga are being discovered and pursued by the West, I think it is important to name some of the cultural assumptions that sit differently in the makeup of thinking in these two cultures.

A caveat: This is my thinking on the subject and is certainly not exhaustible. I am also choosing to speak these differences in broad generalities and to the cultural mix of religion, philosophy, and secular coloring that seems to blend itself into certain contexts. What I see:

West	East
The Pursuit of Attaining	The Pursuit of Letting Go
Morality~Right & Wrong	Ethics~Cause & Effect
Either/Or Thinking	Both/And Thinking
Rules & Answers	Questions & Experiments
Mistakes = Failure	Mistakes = Living

My hope is that we can begin to ask ourselves some very basic questions about our possible unexamined beliefs and assumptions, and this contemplation will take us closer to being impacted by new ideas and bring us a deeper understanding of yogic ethics.

Because we are Spirit hanging out in this body, there is nothing missing that we have to find or gain. Everything we need is already inside of us. Practicing these guidelines is a practice of letting go of limited beliefs and limiting habits that hold us captive to the untruth of our helplessness and despair. Much like peeling away the layers of an onion, we are invited to peel away the beliefs and systems that no longer serve us in living the fullness of our humanity.

Joy does not belong to the world of happiness that advertisers show us. It can not be bought or accomplished, nor is it dependent on external things. External things change; it is their nature to do so. We experience waves of happiness that come with obtaining things, but we also experience waves of sorrow when these things don't do what we want them to. Seeking happiness can only give us the up and down ride of a roller coaster, first we're up, then we plummet down, only to begin the slow ride over again. When we fully embrace our wholeness, we can stop going after things and simply begin to let go of things instead.

To appreciate fully the concept of our wholeness, those of us who have been raised in the United States need to realize the depth to which we have been cultured in the mode of attaining. We have been taught that there is always one more thing that lies outside of us that we need to obtain in order to feel complete. And then one more thing after that. This is knowledge that advertisers take full advantage of and is why we can so easily find ourselves with way too much stuff, and worn out trying to get it. We have, often without paying attention, hoped that one more thing would complete us. We can even find ourselves doing our spirituality as something to be achieved, instead of something we already are.

As you begin to let go of the layers of limits and illusions you have cloaked yourself in, these ten guidelines will meet you at each level of your development. They will reveal new aspects of themselves to you as well as deeper and richer meanings. Much like stocking your shelves with an endless supply of food that can't possibly be eaten at once, these precepts will begin to slowly reveal their secrets to you, and much as an intimate relationship does, they will continue to nourish you and surprise you.

These jewels are not a moral positioning with hard and fast rules. They will not tell you what to believe or what to seek in your life for your own fulfillment. Instead they will equip you to meet each situation with flexibility, understanding, and wisdom. They will give you tools to live more simply, to create less disturbance in your life, and to clear the clutter. Once you have freed up the space, you can listen to the deep longings within and ponder the significant questions of your life.

Whether consciously or unconsciously, we often fall under the spell of the "American Dream." Somehow we have been led to believe that if we do the "right" things, life will bless us with happiness and nice things; when things don't go as intended, we can feel like a failure. The reality of this physical realm is that it is made up of opposites, much like a quarter consists of heads and tails. Only heads, no quarter. Only happiness, no life. Living skillfully does not mean that things go the way we want them to; it means that we are equipped to gracefully meet whatever life greets us with. Hollywood endings are only half of the story.

Rather than the right and wrong of morality, these

guidelines look at life through the eyes of cause and effect. This simply means watching our actions closely and discovering what works and what doesn't. If we get the intended results, continue the action; if not, change the action. Horst Rechelbacher, founder of Aveda Corporation, Intelligent Nutrients, and HMR Enterprises, states in his book *Alivelihood* that he owes much of the vast success of his life to the daily tracking of cause and effect. Horst has gone from a life of poverty in Hungary to become an icon of successful entrepreneurialism in sync with environmental ethics.

Following yoga's jewels takes curiosity and a spirit of adventure. We get to create experiments and track which experiments get the intended results and which don't. From this viewpoint, all of our participation in life is a success because everything we have done gives us valuable information. We are the scientist and our life is the laboratory. As with all scientific experiments, "failure" is a sign of forward movement. And we can be excited by what we don't know and have yet to discover.

The creativity and spontaneity of being able to move mistakes in a forward direction can be illustrated by a story. In my college days, I was a beauty queen candidate. As a remembrance, I was given an autographed rubber football that marked the event. Although I am embarrassed to admit it now, I kept this football for many years, because it made me feel good. When my sons were young, they got a hold of this football and decided to engage in some hands-on ball playing. As a result, the rubber skin of the football was torn in many places. I was not happy.

Then my sons did something I will never forget.

They painstakingly masking-taped the torn football and then painted these words onto the newly repaired football: World's Best Mom. My children understood intuitively the creativity these jewels invite us into. Rather than bask in regrets, guilt, or shame, they turned a "mistake" into such a loving action that it still touches my heart many years later. Wouldn't it be amazing if all of us knew how to take each moment of our life, mistakes and all, and live this creatively? These guidelines can show us how. ℘

Appendix II

The Fruits of the Practice

I am always fascinated when a fresh, new idea seems to hit human consciousness everywhere at once. It is almost like we, as a race, suddenly grew up and were ready to take in a new framework for understanding ourselves. I know this is true when the idea simultaneously appears in various books, and even finds its way onto a bumper sticker. This quote by Jacquelyn Small is an example of an idea, previously unheard of, hitting en masse:

We are not human beings trying to be spiritual;
we are spiritual beings trying to be human.

This statement is quite profound as it shifts the direction of our eyes from looking upward to the heavens to focusing on our humanity here on earth. The question becomes how do we live within the limits of a body and a place and a time? How do we get along with others and share the resources? How do we walk into the fullness of our humanity, creating and enjoying the many opportunities we have to experience life in all its forms, and having as much delight in life as is possible? How do we become skilled and masterful in our humanity?

In the practice of these ethical guidelines, we are steadily taken from self-centeredness to the perfection of humanness in its fullest expression.

Perfection of each Yama brings:

Nonviolence ~ An aura of peace that protects self and other

Truth ~ Spoken words will always come true

Nonstealing ~ Abundance

Nonexcess ~ Great vitality

Nonpossessiveness ~ Knowledge of experience

Perfection of each Niyama brings:

Purity ~ Clarity

Contentment ~ Joy

Self-Discipline ~ Refinement

Self-Study ~ Freedom

Surrender ~ Harmony

❦

Resources

Life is Your Resource

Silly movies, autobiographies of great people, scriptures and teachings of all religions, and the encounters of an ordinary day all have something to say to us.

When we open our eyes and see everything as an opportunity to explore and to learn, nothing becomes insignificant in its ability to teach us and to grow us. ✧

About the Author

Deborah's Bio

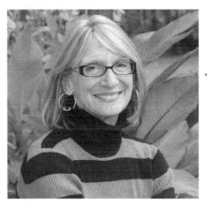

Deborah Adele holds master's degrees in both Liberal Studies and Theology & Religious Studies. An ERYT500, she carries yoga certifications in Kundalini yoga, Hatha yoga, Yoga Therapy, and Meditation. She is also trained as a Gestalt practitioner and a Somatic Educator. For over 14 years, Deborah brought her combined knowledge of business and her in-depth knowledge of yoga philosophy to build Yoga North, now a thriving yoga center. Currently she is writing, teaching, consulting, and engaging her own personal practice.

Deborah worked for three years as a consultant with a firm out of Boulder, Colorado, where she combined the concept of body and breath with organizational development skills to improve leadership and management in various businesses around the country. She wrote a regular wellness column for the Duluth News Tribune and has authored two CD's, *The Art of Relaxation* and *The Practice of Meditation*. Deborah currently owns Adele & Associates, a company whose goal is to increase clarity, productivity, and right-living in individuals and systems. Deborah is a keen and innovative thinker, and, in whatever venue she finds herself, consistently uses her knowledge and training to support others in living a life imbued with balance, clarity, and well-being.

In addition to her business and yoga experience, Deborah has made several trips to India for study and exploration. She feels it is important to continually ask ourselves the question, "What does it mean to be human?" by putting ourselves in places we can be challenged and changed, by telling ourselves the truth, and by sitting in some form of prayer, meditation, or reflection daily.

Deborah currently resides in Duluth with her husband Doug, a Lutheran minister, where their conversations around spirituality remain lively. Her life is enriched by their two sons and four grandchildren.

Deborah's Other Products & Services

Deborah's Other Products

Deborah has authored two CD's, *The Practice of Meditation* and *The Art of Relaxation* to share her love of looking within as a tool to find meaning and to come to greater understanding of the Self.

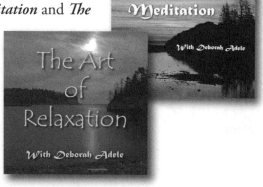

Deborah's Other Services

In addition to authoring a best selling yoga book and two CD's, Deborah offers direct teaching for groups and individuals. Deborah's facilitation leaves participants with a dynamic combination of hope, inspiration, and practical knowledge.

Some of the topics for workshops, keynotes, consultations, teacher trainings, and in depth study programs include:

- Creating Harmony with the Yamas
- Cultivating the Inner Life with the Niyamas
- Pigs Eat Wolves:
    Having a Conversation with your Shadow
- The Whys, Whats and Hows of Meditation
- The Mind: Where Entanglement and Freedom Meet
- The Kleshas: A Yoga Perspective on Suffering
- Freeing the Body's Habits through Somatic Education
- Finding Wellness in Body, Mind, and Spirit
- Beliefs: Leading an Examined Life

Contact Deborah

To learn more about Deborah, keep up with her blog, or see what else she has to offer, visit DeborahAdele.com. You can also contact Deborah directly at Deborah@DeborahAdele.com. ๛

A Note to the Reader:

I wish you richest blessings as you become a more skilled participant in the living of your life. May new possibilities and untold joy surprise you daily.

~D.A.